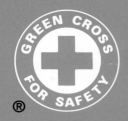

National Safety Council

Bloodborne Pathogens

Second Edition

Editorial, Sales, and Customer Service Offices

Jones and Bartlett Publishers
40 Tall Pine Drive, Sudbury, MA 01776
508•443•5000, 1•800•832•0034
Internet: http://www.jbpub.com/nsc/, email: nsc@jbpub.com

Jones and Bartlett Publishers International
Barb House, Barb Mews
London W6 7PA, UK

Library of Congress Cataloging-in-Publication Data

Bloodborne pathogens / National Safety Council. — 2nd ed.
    p.   cm.
    Includes index.
    ISBN 0-7637-0229-3
    1. Bloodborne infections—Prevention.   I. National Safety
Council.
    RA642.B56B56   1997
    614.4—dc21   96-47085
                                     CIP

The information presented in this book is based on the most recent recommendations of responsible
medical/industrial sources. The National Safety Council, the authors and the publisher, however, make no
guarantee as to, and assume no responsibility for, correctness, sufficiency, or completeness of such information or recommendations. Other or additional measures may be required under particular circumstances.

The OSHA Bloodborne Pathogens Standard is an evolving standard. The authors are in no way
responsible for changes made in the standard after the printing of this text. Annual training is
required to keep up with changes in the standard.

Chief Executive Officer ■ Clayton E. Jones
Emergency Care Editor ■ Tracy Murphy
Production Administrator ■ Anne S. Noonan
Manufacturing Manager ■ Dana L. Cerrito
Editorial Production Service ■ Books By Design, Inc.
Typesetting and Pre-press ■ Pre-Press Company, Inc.
Cover Design ■ Marshall Henrichs
Printing and Binding ■ Banta Company

Printed in the United States of America
00 99 98 97 96   10 9 8 7 6 5 4 3 2 1

Table of Contents

Acknowledgments

Principal Authors

Karen Commeau, R.N.C.
Technical Writer
Systems Consulting
    Company, Inc.
Portland, ME

Mark Jackson, M.D.
Director of Student Health
    Services
Cutler Health Center
University of Maine
Orono, ME

Sally McKinnon, B.S.N.
Associate for Clinical
    Management
Chief of Ambulance Service
Coordinator for HAZMAT
    Communications and
    Bloodborne Pathogens
    Standard
Cutler Health Center
University of Maine
Orono, ME

Principal Reviewers

Sonny Barclift
Arizona Chapter, National Safety
    Council
Phoenix, AZ

Peggy Baum
Health and Safety Administrator
University of Maine
Orono, ME

Carol Bufton
Minnesota Safety Council
St. Paul, MN

Richard Cooper
SEMTA
Rye, NH

Betty Jane Evans
Dade County Citizens Safety Council
Miami, FL

Kay Farrell
Safety and Health Council of
    Greater Omaha
Omaha, NE

Patty Fernandez
Tampa Area Safety Council
Tampa, FL

First Aid and CPR Advisory
    Committee
New Jersey State Safety Council
Cranford, NJ

Donna Gates
Health Care and Nursing Consultants
Lexington, KY

David A. Gibbs
Safety Compliance Specialist
State of Maine
Bureau of Labor Standards
Augusta, Maine

Grant Gould
Safety Consultants
Fair Oaks, CA

Lynne Lamstein, M.S.I.H.
Occupational Health Specialist
State of Maine
Department of Labor
Bureau of Labor Standards
Augusta, Maine

Mary Olszewski
Safety Council of Maryland
Baltimore, MD

Jodi Rupe
Texas Safety Association
Austin, TX

Donna Siegfried
First Aid Institute
National Safety Council
Itasca, Illinois

Michael E. Szczygiel
Medevac Medical Services, Inc.
Topeka, KS

Alton Thygerson, Ph.D.
Brigham Young University
Provo, Utah

About the National Safety Council Program

Congratulations on selecting the National Safety Council! You join good company, as the National Safety Council has successfully trained over 2 million people worldwide. The National Safety Council's training network of nearly 10,000 instructors at over 2,500 sites worldwide has established the National Safety Council programs as the standard by which all others are judged.

In setting the standards, the National Safety Council has worked in close cooperation with hundreds of national and international organizations, thousands of corporations, thousands of leading educators, dozens of leading medical organizations, and hundreds of state and local governmental agencies. Their collective input has helped create programs that stand alone in quality. Consider just a few of the National Safety Council's current collaborations:

World's Leading Medical Organizations

The National Safety Council is currently working with both the American Academy of Orthopaedic Surgeons (AAOS) and the Wilderness Medical Society (WMS) to help bring innovative, new training programs to the marketplace. The National Safety Council and the AAOS are developing a new First Responder program and the National Safety Council and the WMS are developing the first-of-its-kind wilderness first aid program.

United States Government

The National Safety Council has developed an innovative computer-based training program for first aid that is currently being used to train United States Postal Service employees.

World's Leading Corporations

Thousands of corporations including Westinghouse, Disney, Exxon, General Motors, Pacific Bell, Ameritech, and U.S. West have selected many of the National Safety Council emergency care programs to train employees.

World's Leading Colleges and Universities

Hundreds of leading colleges and universities are working closely with the National Safety Council to fully develop and implement the Internet Initiative that will establish the National Safety Council as the leading on-line provider of emergency care programs.

Most importantly, in selecting the National Safety Council programs, you can feel confident that the programs are accepted and approved worldwide.

You can rely on the National Safety Council. Founded in 1913, the National Safety Council is dedicated to protecting life, promoting health, and reducing accidental death. For more than 80 years, the National Safety Council has been the world's leading authority on safety/injury education.

National Safety Council

1

Introduction

■ What Is the OSHA Bloodborne Pathogens Standard? ■ Who Needs This Manual? ■
■ Why Do I Need This Manual? ■ Meeting OSHA Standards ■

What Is the OSHA Bloodborne Pathogens Standard?

The 1991 OSHA (Occupational Safety and Health Administration) regulations include a section specific to bloodborne pathogens, section 1910.1030. This standard provides requirements for employers to follow to ensure employee safety with regard to occupational exposure to bloodborne pathogens.

Who Needs This Manual?

Any employee who has potential for occupational exposure to blood or other potentially infectious materials (OPIM) is required to receive training according to the bloodborne pathogens standard. The following job classifications may be associated with tasks that have occupational exposure to blood or OPIM, but the standard is not limited to employees in these positions.

- Physicians, physicians' assistants, nurses, nurse practitioners, and other health care employees in clinics and physicians' offices
- Employees of clinical and diagnostic laboratories
- Housekeepers in health care facilities
- Personnel in hospital laundries or commercial laundries that service health care or public safety institutions
- Tissue bank personnel
- Employees in blood banks and plasma centers who collect, transport, and test blood, Free-standing clinic employees (for instance, hemodialysis clinics, urgent care clinics, health maintenance organization (HMO) clinics, and family planning clinics)
- Employees in clinics in industrial, educational, and correctional facilities (for example, those who collect blood, and clean and dress wounds)
- Employees assigned to provide emergency first aid
- Dentists, dental hygienists, dental assistants, and dental laboratory technicians
- Staff of institutions for the developmentally disabled
- Hospice employees

- Home health care workers
- Staff of nursing homes and long-term care facilities
- Employees of funeral homes and mortuaries
- HIV and HBV research laboratory and production facility workers
- Employees handling regulated waste
- Medical equipment service and repair personnel
- Emergency medical technicians, paramedics, and other emergency medical service providers
- Firefighters, law enforcement personnel, and correctional officers

Note: Good Samaritan Acts are not covered under the standard.

Why Do I Need This Manual?

This manual provides a written reference for your personal use during both this session of bloodborne pathogens training and later, at the worksite.

It also offers exercises at the end of each chapter to help you check what you have learned and how it applies to your job.

Meeting OSHA Standards

The 1991 OSHA Bloodborne Pathogens Standard mandates annual training for all employees with occupational exposure to blood or OPIM.

A good rule of thumb to determine whether your job requires exposure to blood or OPIM is to ask yourself if you would be reprimanded for not helping someone who is bleeding, or for failing to open packages that might contain blood or OPIM.

The training must be offered at no cost to the employee during regular work hours.

We encourage all employees to receive the training in any site where exposure to blood or OPIM is possible. Employees whose duties do not require exposure to blood or OPIM also should be made aware of worksite hazards as well as the meaning of the terms biohazard, red bags, labeling and disposal of regulated waste to protect themselves from inadvertent exposures. The standards include the potential

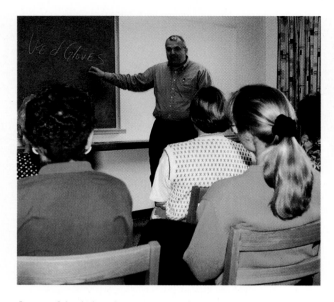

Annual training is necessary to ensure employee safety.

for exposure, not just actual exposure. For example, a front desk receptionist may not have an actual exposure to a bleeding patient, but the potential for exposure may exist.

This training must be presented in language appropriate in content and vocabulary to the educational and literacy level of the employee. If employees are only proficient in a foreign language, training must be presented in that foreign language.

The employer must provide additional training when there is a change in the tasks and procedures that affects the employees' occupational exposure.

The training program must provide employees with the following:

1. An accessible copy of the regulatory text (Appendix B) and an explanation of its contents (this manual)

2. A general explanation of the epidemiology and symptoms of bloodborne disease (Chapter 2)

3. An explanation of the modes of transmission of bloodborne pathogens (Chapter 9)

4. An explanation of the employer's Exposure Control Plan and the means by which the employee can obtain a copy of the written plan (supplied by your company directly or through the instructor)

5. An explanation of the appropriate methods for recognizing tasks and other activities that may involve exposure to blood and other potentially infectious materials (Chapter 10)

6. An explanation of the use and limitations of methods that will prevent or reduce exposure including appropriate engineering controls, work practices, and personal protective equipment (Chapters 3, 4, and 6)

7. Information on the types, proper use, location, removal, handling, decontamination, and disposal of personal protective equipment (Chapter 7)

8. An explanation of the basis for selection of personal protective equipment (Chapter 6)

9. Information on the Hepatitis B vaccine, including information on its efficacy, safety, method of administration, the benefits of being vaccinated, and that the vaccine and vaccination will be offered free of charge to employees covered by the standard (Chapter 5)

10. Information on the appropriate actions to take and persons to contact in an emergency involving blood or other potentially infectious materials (Chapter 11)

11. An explanation of the procedure to follow if an exposure incident occurs including the method of reporting the incident and the medical follow-up that will be made available (Chapter 11)

12. Information on the post-exposure evaluation and follow-up that the employer is required to provide for the employee following an exposure incident (Chapter 11)

13. An explanation of the signs, labels, and/or color-coding required (Chapter 8)

14. An opportunity for interactive questions and answers with the person conducting the training session (during and after training session)

Note: Failure to meet the standards may result in fines to the employer.

The Ryan White Act

The CDC is in the process of preparing the final list of diseases required by the passage of the Public Law 101-381, the Ryan White Comprehensive AIDS Resources Emergency Act. The Act creates a notification system for emergency response employees listed as police, fire, and EMS, who are exposed to diseases such as *M. tuberculosis,* Hepatitis B or C, and HIV.

Name _____ Course _____ Date _____

■ ACTIVITY 1 ■
Training Requirements

Mark each statement true (T) or false (F).

1. _____ Training on OSHA bloodborne pathogens regulations must be provided annually.

2. _____ It is the employee's responsibility to seek appropriate training on bloodborne pathogens.

3. _____ An employer may decide not to provide training if it is not cost effective.

4. _____ Additional training is required if there is a change in the tasks or procedures that affect employee occupational exposure.

5. _____ Training is performed during regular work hours.

6. _____ Employees must be given a copy of the regulations and an explanation of their contents.

7. _____ The training program must include information on what to do in the event of an occupational exposure to bloodborne pathogens.

8. _____ After training, employees should be familiar with the symptoms of bloodborne disease.

2
Bloodborne Pathogens

■ What Are Bloodborne Pathogens? ■ Hepatitis B Infection ■
■ Human Immunodeficiency Virus (HIV) ■

Learning Objective

You will be able to explain the transmission, course, and effects of bloodborne pathogens.

What Are Bloodborne Pathogens?

- Bloodborne pathogens are disease-causing microorganisms that may be present in human blood. They may be transmitted with any exposure to blood or OPIM.
- Two pathogens of significance are Hepatitis B Virus (HBV) and Human Immunodeficiency Virus (HIV).
- A number of bloodborne diseases other than HIV and HBV exist, such as Hepatitis C, Hepatitis D, and syphilis.

Hepatitis B Infection

- Hepatitis B Virus (HBV) is one of five viruses that causes illness directly affecting the liver.
- Hepatitis B Virus is a major cause of viral hepatitis for which prevention is possible through immunization. Hepatitis results in swelling, soreness, and loss of normal functions of the liver.
- The symptoms of Hepatitis B include weakness, fatigue, anorexia, nausea, abdominal pain, fever, and headache.
- Jaundice, a yellow discoloration of the skin, is a symptom that may develop.
- Hepatitis B may have no symptoms and therefore may not be diagnosed.
- A person's blood will test positive for the HBV surface antigen within 2 to 6 weeks after symptoms of the illness develop.
- Approximately 85 percent of patients recover in 6 to 8 weeks.
- A major source of HBV is chronic carriers. Chronic carriers will have the antigen present at all times and can unwittingly transmit the disease to sus-

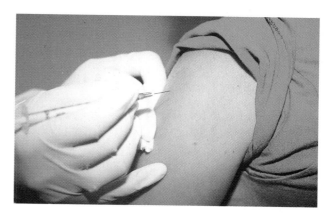

Immunization against HBV is possible.

ceptible persons through needle, or other penetrating injury, and intimate contact.
- Chronic active hepatitis may be the consequence of a problem with the immune system that prevents the complete destruction of virus-infected liver cells.

Key Facts

- Approximately 8,700 health care workers contract Hepatitis B each year, and about 200 will die.
- Cases of acute Hepatitis B infection have increased 37 percent from 1979 to 1989.
- It is estimated that 200,000 to 300,000 new infections occurred annually from 1980 to 1991.
- It is estimated that 1 to 1.25 million persons in the United States have chronic hepatitis B and are potentially infectious to others.

Key Facts

- It is estimated that 1 in 250 persons in the United States is infected with HIV.
- There are at least 65 case reports of health care workers whose HIV infection is associated with occupational exposure.
- According to the World Health Organization, 10 to 12 million people around the world are infected with HIV.
- Approximately 200,000 AIDS patients have been reported to the Centers for Disease Control thus far, 84 of whom are health care workers with no other identified reason for infection.
- The Centers for Disease Control reports that prisons have a higher incidence of HIV infection than any other public institution. In a 1990 survey, 5.8 percent of prison inmates were found to be infected.

Human Immunodeficiency Virus (HIV)

- Human Immunodeficiency Virus (HIV) is a virus that infects immune system T_4 blood cells in humans and renders them less effective in preventing disease.
- It is the virus identified as responsible for Acquired Immunodeficiency Syndrome (AIDS).
- Symptoms of HIV might include night sweats, weight loss, fever, fatigue, gland pain or swelling, and muscle or joint pain.
- People with HIV may feel fine and not be aware that they have been exposed to HIV for as much as 8 to 10 years.
- It may take as long as a year for a blood test to become positive for HIV antibodies. Therefore, more than one test may be required to determine if a person has been infected.

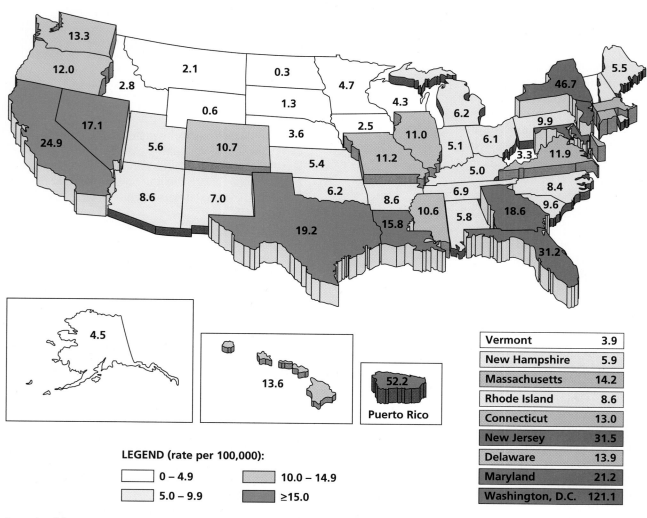

State	Rate
Vermont	3.9
New Hampshire	5.9
Massachusetts	14.2
Rhode Island	8.6
Connecticut	13.0
New Jersey	31.5
Delaware	13.9
Maryland	21.2
Washington, D.C.	121.1

LEGEND (rate per 100,000):

- 0 – 4.9
- 5.0 – 9.9
- 10.0 – 14.9
- ≥15.0

Acquired Immunodeficiency Syndrome (AIDS). Cases per 100,000 population. Reported to CDC by state, United States, 1990.

Name _____ Course _____ Date _____

■ ACTIVITY 1 ■
Bloodborne Pathogens

Match the statement with either HBV or HIV.

1. _____ It may take up to a year for a blood test to become positive, and more than one test may be required.

2. _____ The symptoms include weakness, fatigue, nausea, and headache.

3. _____ Approximately 85 percent of patients recover in 6 to 8 weeks.

4. _____ A virus that infects immune system blood cells in humans.

5. _____ One of five viruses that affect the liver.

■ ACTIVITY 2 ■
Worksite Evaluation

1. Identify two places at your worksite where exposure to blood or OPIM could occur.

_____

_____

_____

_____

2. Explain an area of your occupation that might expose you to bloodborne pathogens.

_____

_____

_____

_____

3
Prevention

■ **Engineering Controls** ■ **Work Practice Controls** ■
■ **Personal Protective Equipment** ■ **Universal Precautions** ■

Learning Objective

You will be able to identify four ways to prevent an exposure incident to bloodborne pathogens.

To minimize exposure to bloodborne pathogens there are four strategies of prevention. These strategies are used in combination to offer you maximum protection.

■ Engineering controls attempt to design safety into the tools and workspace organization. An example is a sharps container.

■ Work practice controls are the use of equipment with engineered protections. An example would be immediately putting contaminated sharps into a sharps container.

■ When occupational exposure remains after using engineering and work practice controls, employers must provide personal protective equipment. Personal protective equipment is used to protect you from contamination of skin, mucous membranes, or puncture wounds.

■ Universal Precautions is a strategy to structure your approach to working with all human blood and certain body fluids. Another method of infection control is called Body Substance Isolation (BSI). This method defines all body fluids and substances as infectious. BSI includes all fluids and materials covered by the standard.

All these strategies combined promote worker safety and provide a safer working environment.

Engineering Controls

Engineering controls are structural or mechanical devices the company provides. Examples include handwashing facilities, eye stations, sharps containers, and biohazard labels.

Work Practice Controls

Work practice controls are the behaviors necessary to use engineering controls effectively. These include, but are not limited to, using sharps containers, using an eye wash station, and washing your hands after removing personal protective equipment.

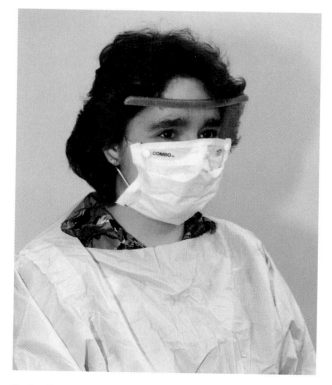

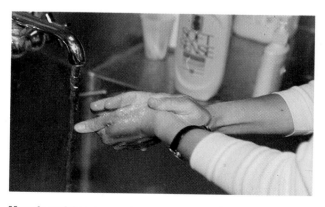

Handwashing is a primary means of prevention.

Protective equipment is provided for your protection.

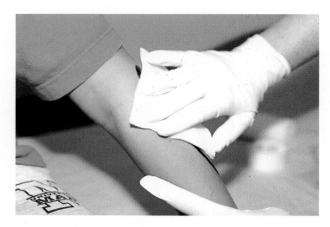

Universal Precautions protect everyone.

Personal Protective Equipment

Personal protective equipment is equipment provided by your employer at no cost to you. It is to your advantage to use this equipment. Report to your supervisor when any equipment is not in working order.

Personal protective equipment includes materials such as latex gloves, masks, aprons, gowns, and face shields.

Universal Precautions

Universal Precautions is the concept that all blood and certain body fluids are to be treated as if contaminated with HIV, HBV, or other bloodborne pathogens.

Body Substance Isolation can be used as an alternative to Universal Precautions. This method treats all fluids and substances as infectious and is acceptable under the standard.

Name _____ Course _____ Date _____

■ ACTIVITY 1 ■
Prevention

There are four strategies recommended by OSHA to protect the employee from an exposure incident to bloodborne pathogens: engineering controls, work practice controls, personal protective equipment, and Universal Precautions. Match the description to the strategy.

1. _____ Materials such as gloves, gowns, masks, and face shields are provided by the employer.

2. _____ The concept that all blood and some body fluids should be treated as if contaminated with HIV and/or HBV.

3. _____ Examples of this strategy include sharps containers, handwashing facilities, eye stations, biohazard waste containers, etc.

4. _____ Employee using gloves while giving an injection.

A. Engineering controls
B. Work practice controls
C. Personal protective equipment
D. Universal Precautions

■ ACTIVITY 2 ■
Prevention Strategies

Choose the best answer.

1. _____ What is the most effective method of preventing transmission of bloodborne pathogens?
A. Gloves and mask
B. Immunization against Hepatitis B Virus
C. Handwashing
D. Eye stations

2. _____ Which of the following was not a method of prevention outlined in the text.
A. Personal protective equipment
B. Universal Precautions
C. Immediately reporting all incidents
D. Work practice controls

4
Universal Precautions

■ Universal Precautions ■ Materials That Require Universal Precautions ■
■ Materials That Do Not Require Universal Precautions ■ Personal Protective Equipment ■

Learning Objective

You will be able to describe the concept of Universal Precautions and explain the materials that require precautions.

Universal Precautions

Universal Precautions is an aggressive, standardized approach to infection control. According to the concept of Universal Precautions, you should treat all human blood and certain body fluids as if they are known to contain HIV, HBV, or other bloodborne pathogens.

Body Substance Isolation

Another method of infection control is called Body Substance Isolation (BSI). This method defines all body fluids and substances as infectious. BSI includes not only the fluids and materials covered by this standard but expands coverage to all body fluids and substances.

BSI is an acceptable alternative to Universal Precautions provided facilities using BSI adhere to all other provisions of this standard.

Materials That Require Universal Precautions

Universal Precautions apply to the following potentially infectious materials:

■ Blood
■ Semen
■ Vaginal secretions
■ Cerebrospinal fluid
■ Synovial fluid
■ Pleural fluid
■ Any body fluid with visible blood
■ Any unidentifiable body fluid
■ Saliva from dental procedures

Materials That Do Not Require Universal Precautions

Universal Precautions do *not* apply to the following body fluids unless they contain visible blood:

■ Feces
■ Nasal secretions
■ Sputum
■ Sweat
■ Tears
■ Urine
■ Vomitus

Personal Protective Equipment

You must use personal protective equipment such as gloves or a mask whenever you might be exposed to blood or OPIM. (See table: Determining the Need for Universal Precautions.)

Determining the Need for Universal Precautions

Incident	Universal Precautions Needed?	Suggested Action
Nurse is going to change dressing on a recent wound.	YES	Nurse should wear latex gloves and/or other personal protective equipment whenever at risk of exposure to blood or potentially infectious materials.
Teacher is approached by young, hysterical student with a bloody nose.	YES	If required to attend to the student, the teacher should reassure child, put on latex gloves and follow the routine procedures at your facility.
An ambulance attendant is called to a home where an elderly gentleman appears to have had a heart attack. The gentleman is conscious and able to speak.	NO	There is no immediate blood or infectious materials, the attendant may need to perform CPR in the event of cardiac or respiratory arrest. **Note:** In the event of cardiac or respiratory arrest, work practice controls and personal protective equipment may be required.
A police officer pulls over a car that has a burned out headlight.	NO	It is unlikely that the police officer will come in contact with blood or potentially infectious materials.
A laboratory worker is testing urine for evidence of infection. The specimen appears to have a trace of blood.	YES	The laboratory worker should be using personal protective equipment whenever dealing with any specimens with visible blood.

Name _____ Course _____ Date _____

■ ACTIVITY 1 ■
Universal Precautions

A. Mark each statement as true (T) or false (F).

1. ____ Universal Precautions applies to human blood and other potentially infectious materials.

2. ____ According to the concept of Universal Precautions, an athlete should wear some sort of personal protective equipment because of possible exposure to another athlete's sweat.

3. ____ Universal Precautions do not apply to urine under any circumstances.

4. ____ Universal Precautions apply to semen under all circumstances.

5. ____ Body substance isolation is an acceptable alternative to Universal Precautions.

B. Choose the best answer.

1. ____ Universal Precautions refers to:
   A. A comprehensive approach to infection control.
   B. Treating all human blood as potentially infectious.
   C. A way to protect you from transmission of bloodborne pathogens.
   D. All of the above.

2. ____ Imagine that you are the teacher in a schoolyard and Charles comes up to you with a bloody knee. What should you do?
   A. Send him to the school nurse.
   B. It's just a scrape, put a bandage on it.
   C. Follow the Exposure Control Plan at your facility.
   D. Have him sit out the recess to remind him to be more careful.

■ ACTIVITY 2 ■
Worksite Evaluation

1. Identify two examples of when Universal Precautions would be needed in your work assignment.

_____

_____

_____

2. What potentially infectious materials do you encounter in your work assignment?

_____

_____

_____

5

Immunization

- Hepatitis B Vaccines ■ Who Should Receive the Vaccine ■
- Contraindications ■ Side Effects of the Vaccine ■

Learning Objective

You will be able to describe the types of Hepatitis B vaccine, their usage, and contraindications.

All people who have routine occupational exposure to blood or other potentially infectious materials have the right to receive the immunization series against Hepatitis B at no personal expense. The standard includes temporary and part-time workers.

Prescreening is not required, and your employer may not make prescreening a requirement for receiving the vaccine. If you choose to have prescreening, the testing must be done at an accredited laboratory.

The standard requires that your employer offer the vaccine to you at a convenient time, during normal work hours. If travel is required away from the worksite, your employer is responsible for that cost. The standard includes temporary and part-time workers.

Your employer cannot require you to use your health insurance to pay for the cost of the vaccine. Your employer cannot require you to pay and then be reimbursed if you remain employed for a specific time. Nor are you required to reimburse your employer for the cost of the vaccine if you leave your job.

You may refuse the series by signing the Hepatitis B vaccine declination form (Appendix C). If you change your mind while still covered under the standard at a later date, you may still receive the vaccine at no cost.

Hepatitis B Vaccines

Recombivax HB is vaccine provided by Merck Sharp & Dohme, or Engerix-B by Smith-Kline, Inc., are the vaccines used to prevent infection with the Hepatitis B Virus. The vaccine is given in three doses over a 6-month period; the first is given at an agreed-on date, the second is given 1 month later, and the third dose is given 5 months after the second dose. The vaccine is administered by needle into a large muscle such as the deltoid in the upper arm.

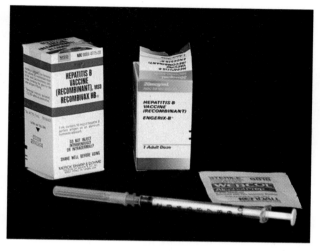

Hepatitis B vaccine is available from a variety of manufacturers.

In persons receiving the vaccine, 87 percent will develop immunity after the second dose of the vaccine, and 96 percent will develop immunity after the third dose.

Who Should Receive the Vaccine

The Hepatitis B vaccine series is recommended for the following groups. This list is suggestive and by no means inclusive.

- Health care personnel
- Custodial staff that have possible exposure to bloodborne pathogens such as those working in health care settings or laboratories
- Dental, medical, and nursing students
- Any personnel exposed to blood or blood products such as laboratory and blood bank personnel
- Lifeguards, firefighters, teachers, police officers, sport team coaches, and trainers

Contraindications

You should not receive the vaccine if you are sensitive to yeast or any other component of the vaccine. Consultation with a physician is required for persons with heart disease, fever, or other illness.

If you are pregnant or breastfeeding an infant, you should consult your physician before receiving the vaccine.

Side Effects of the Vaccine

The side effects of the vaccine are minimal and may include localized swelling, pain, bruising, or redness at the injection site. The most common systemic reactions include flu-like symptoms such as fatigue, weakness, headache, fever, or malaise.

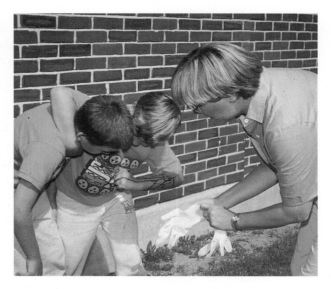

Hepatitis B vaccine is recommended for anyone with occupational exposure to bloodborne pathogens.

■ DECISION FOR HEPATITIS B IMMUNIZATION ■

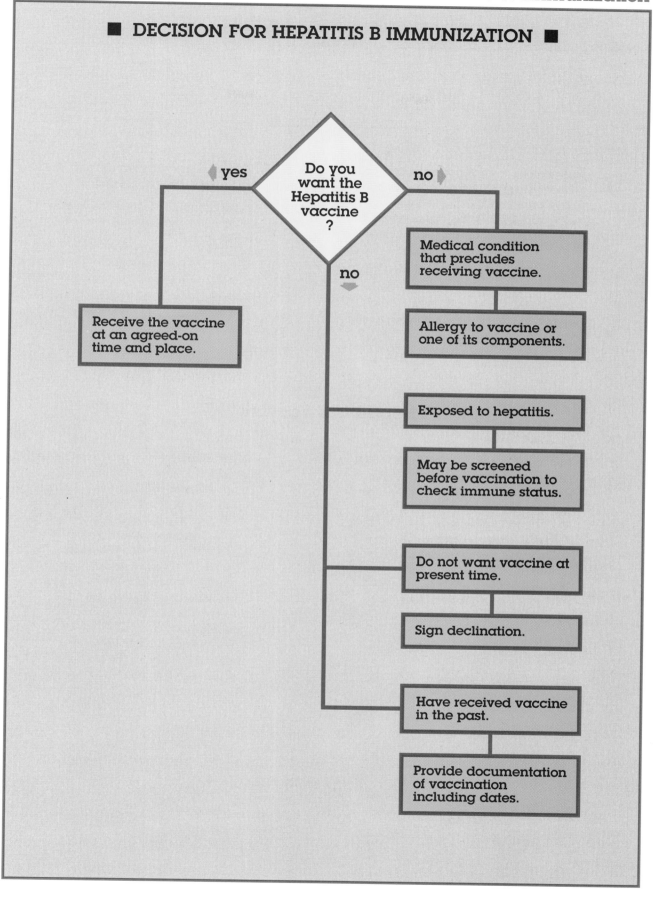

Do you want the Hepatitis B vaccine ?

yes

no

no

Receive the vaccine at an agreed-on time and place.

Medical condition that precludes receiving vaccine.

Allergy to vaccine or one of its components.

Exposed to hepatitis.

May be screened before vaccination to check immune status.

Do not want vaccine at present time.

Sign declination.

Have received vaccine in the past.

Provide documentation of vaccination including dates.

Name _____ Course _____ Date _____

■ ACTIVITY 1 ■
Immunization

Mark each statement true (T) or false (F).

1. _____ All persons covered under the OSHA Bloodborne Pathogens Standard who have a routine exposure to blood or other potentially infectious materials may receive the Hepatitis B vaccine at no personal expense.

2. _____ Even if an employee signs a waiver refusing the immunization, the employer must provide the Hepatitis B vaccine if the employee requests it while still covered under the standard.

3. _____ Hepatitis B vaccine is given in a six dose series over a 12-month period.

4. _____ Because the side effects of the vaccine are so minor, most people choose to receive it.

■ ACTIVITY 2 ■
Hepatitis B Vaccine

Choose the best answer.

1. _____ Hepatitis B vaccine is available to all employees covered by the OSHA standard. The employee is responsible for:
   A. The cost of the vaccine only.
   B. The cost of the vaccine and the office visit to receive the injection.
   C. Showing up at the site at an agreed-on time.
   D. The cost of the office visit to the doctor's office. The employer is responsible for the cost of the vaccine.

2. _____ May an employee who is covered under the OSHA Bloodborne Pathogens Standard refuse the Hepatitis B vaccine?
   A. Yes, but only for medical reasons. The person must have a letter written by a physician stating the reasons.
   B. Yes, but the person must sign the waiver form, have a medical reason for refusing, or have already received it.
   C. No, under the standard you must receive the vaccine for your own protection.
   D. Yes, but once an employee has refused the vaccine the person is never eligible to receive the vaccine again at the expense of the employer.

6

Exposure Control

■ **Engineering and Work Practice Controls** ■ **Personal Protective Equipment** ■
■ **Limited Exceptions to Using Personal Protective Equipment** ■

Learning Objective

You will be able to describe the controls that reduce exposure to bloodborne pathogens.

Engineering and Work Practice Controls

OSHA requires safety to be engineered into the tools and workspaces. Work practice controls are the required behaviors necessary to take full advantage of the engineered controls. Both are used to eliminate or minimize exposure to bloodborne pathogens. If risk of occupational exposure exists even when engineering and work practice controls are instituted, workers must use personal protective equipment for their protection and safety.

Your employer is responsible for the full cost of instituting engineering and work practice controls. Engineering controls must be examined and maintained or replaced on a regular schedule to ensure effectiveness and safety. This task may be assigned to you by your employer. It is a violation of the standard if effective monitoring does not take place.

Handwashing and Handwashing Facilities

Employers are required to provide handwashing facilities that are readily accessible to all employees. The standard specifies that the handwashing facility must be situated so that employees do not have to use stairs, doorways, and corridors, which might result in environmental surface contamination.

If the provision of handwashing facilities is not feasible (such as in an ambulance or police car), the employer must provide either an appropriate antiseptic hand cleanser with clean cloth or paper towels, or antiseptic towelettes. If you use antiseptic hand cleansers or towelettes, you must wash your hands with soap and warm water as soon as possible after contact with blood or OPIM.

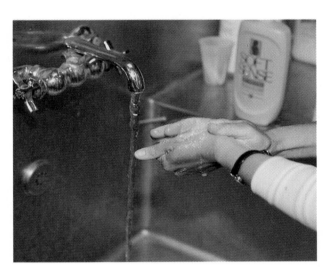

Handwashing is a primary means of preventing transmission of bloodborne pathogens.

Groups that may use alternative washing methods such as antiseptic hand cleaners and towelettes are ambulance-based paramedics, EMTs, firefighters, police, and mobile blood collection personnel. All groups must wash with soap and warm water as soon as possible after contact with blood or OPIM.

Employers shall ensure that employees wash hands and any other contaminated skin with soap and warm water (or flush mucous membranes with water) as soon as possible following contact with blood or OPIM. Employees must wash hands and skin surfaces after the removal of gloves or other personal protective equipment.

Work Practice Controls

All procedures involving blood or OPIM shall be performed in such a way as to minimize or eliminate splashing, spraying, splattering, and generation of droplets of these substances.

Mouth pipetting or suctioning of blood or OPIM is prohibited. This procedure should *never* occur unless it is part of a specialized procedure such as DeLee suctioning. However, even then there must be a one-way

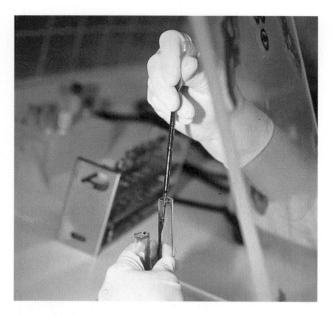

All procedures should be performed to minimize splashing.

valve between the patient and the practitioner.

Eating, drinking, smoking, applying cosmetics or lip balm, and handling contact lenses is *prohibited* in work areas where there is a reasonable likelihood of occupational exposure to blood or OPIM. Hand cream is not considered a cosmetic and is permitted under the standard. It should be noted, however, that some petroleum-based hand creams can adversely affect glove integrity.

Food or drink must not be kept in refrigerators, freezers, shelves, cabinets, countertops, or benches where blood or OPIM is present.

You must remove all personal protective equipment and wash your hands prior to leaving the work area. To prevent contamination of employee eating areas do not enter eating or break areas while wearing personal protective equipment.

Contaminated Needles or Sharps

OSHA defines contaminated sharps as any contaminated object that can penetrate the skin, including, but not limited to, needles, scalpels, broken capillary tubes, and exposed ends of dental wires.

Contaminated needles or other contaminated sharps must not be bent, recapped, or removed unless it can be demonstrated that no alternative is feasible or that such action is required by a specific medical procedure. If a procedure requires shearing or breaking of needles, this procedure must be specified in the company's Exposure Control Plan.

Needle removal or recapping needles must be accomplished through a one-handed technique or the use of a mechanical device. (See Skill Scan on One-Handed Technique.)

Reusable sharps must be placed in clearly labeled, puncture-resistant, leakproof containers immediately or as soon as possible after use until they can be reprocessed. *Never* blindly reach into a container containing contaminated sharps.

Personal Protective Equipment

Personal protective equipment is specialized clothing or equipment worn or used by you for protection against hazard. This includes equipment such as latex gloves, gowns, aprons, face shields, masks, eye protection, laboratory coats, CPR microshield, and resuscitation bags.

Whenever you need to wear a face mask, you must also wear eye protection. If you are wearing your personal glasses, you must use side shields and plan to decontaminate your glasses and side shields according to the schedule determined by your employer.

Personal protective equipment is acceptable if it prevents blood or OPIM from contaminating work clothes, street clothes, undergarments, skin, eyes, mouth, or other mucous membranes.

Your employer is responsible for providing personal protective equipment at no expense to you. Equipment must be provided in appropriate sizes and placed within easy reach for all employees.

Hypoallergenic gloves, glove liners, powderless gloves, or other similar alternatives shall be provided to you if you are allergic to gloves normally provided.

Your employer is responsible for cleaning, laundering, disposal, and replacement of personal protective equipment at no charge to you.

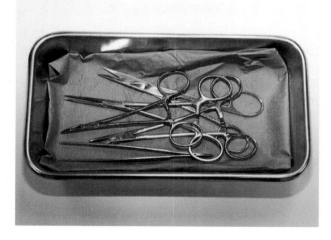

Using caution with reusable sharps can prevent injury and disease.

- Studies have shown that gloves provide a barrier, but that neither vinyl nor latex procedure gloves are completely impermeable.

- Disinfecting agents may cause deterioration of the glove material; washing with surfactants could result in wicking or enhanced penetration of liquids into the glove via undetected pores, thereby transporting blood and OPIM into contact with the hand. For this reason, disposable (single-use) gloves may not be washed and reused.

- Certain solutions such as iodine may cause discoloration of gloves without affecting their integrity and function.

If blood or OPIM contaminates your clothing, you must remove it as soon as feasible and place it in an appropriately designated area or container.

If a pullover scrub or shirt becomes contaminated, you must remove it in such a way as to avoid contact with the outer surface—for example, rolling up the garment as it is pulled toward the head for removal. However, if the blood penetrates the scrub or shirt and contaminates the inner surface, the penetration itself would constitute an exposure. If the scrub or shirt cannot be removed without contamination of the face, it is recommended that the shirt be cut and removed.

If your personal protective equipment has been penetrated by blood or OPIM, it is recommended that you check your body for cuts or scrapes or other non-intact skin when removing your equipment.

You must remove all personal protective equipment before leaving the work area to prevent transmission of bloodborne pathogens to co-workers in other departments and family, and to prevent contamination of environmental surfaces.

Limited Exceptions to Using Personal Protective Equipment

There are a few exceptions to the use of personal protective equipment when the use of such equipment would prevent the proper delivery of health care or public safety services, or would pose an increased hazard to the personal safety of the worker. Examples of such situations could include:

- A sudden change in patient status such as when an apparently stable patient unexpectedly begins to hemorrhage profusely, putting the patient's life in immediate jeopardy
- A firefighter rescuing an individual who is not breathing from a burning building discovers that the resuscitation equipment is lost or damaged and must administer CPR
- A bleeding suspect unexpectedly attacks a police officer with a knife, threatening the safety of the officer and/or co-workers.

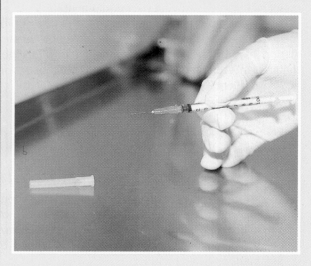

Needle removal or recapping must be accomplished through the use of a mechanical device or one-handed technique to prevent puncture wounds.

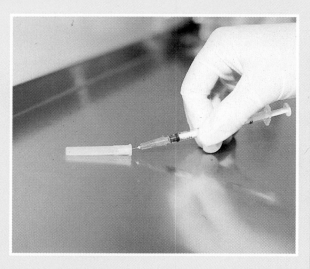

The one-handed technique uses a nearby wall or heavy object to stabilize the needle cover.

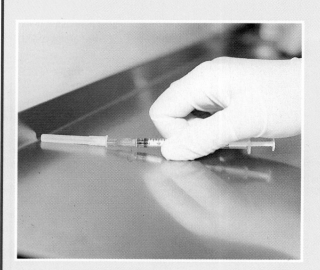

Using one hand, gently slide the needle into the needle cover.

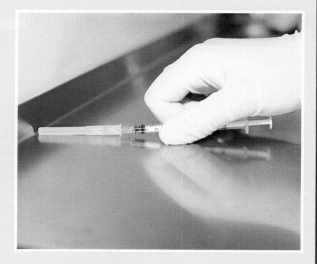

Using the wall as support, apply gentle pressure to secure the needle cover. Dispose of the needle and syringe in nearest sharps container.

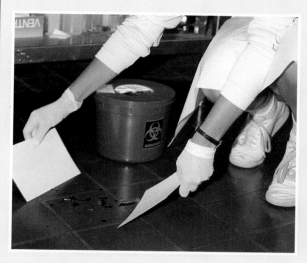

When cleaning up broken glass, wear gloves and/or other personal protective equipment.

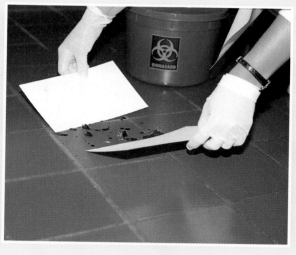

Do not clean up broken glass with your hands. Instead use a dust pan and brush, cardboard (as shown), or tongs.

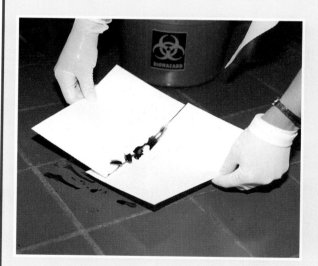

Vacuum cleaners are prohibited for the cleaning up of broken glass.

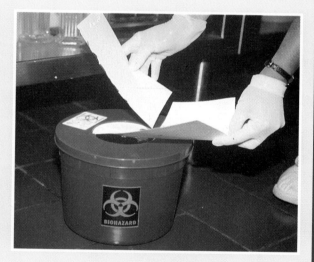

Broken glass must be placed in an appropriate sharps container. Placing broken glass in a plastic bag may put others at risk for exposure.

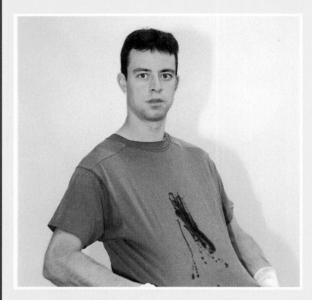

If a pull-over shirt becomes contaminated, you must remove it in such a way as to avoid contact with the outer surface.

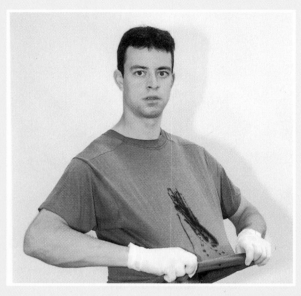

Rolling the garment as it is pulled toward the head will decrease the chance of contact with the contaminated area.

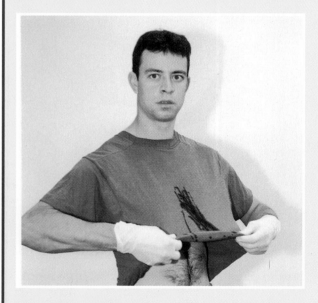

After rolling up the shirt, carefully pull it over the head to avoid contact with the face or mucous membranes.

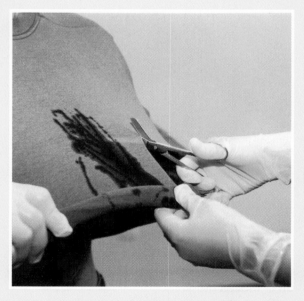

If the shirt cannot be removed without contamination, it is recommended that the shirt be cut off.

Name _____ Course _____ Date _____

■ ACTIVITY 1 ■
Exposure Control

A. Mark each statement true (T) or false (F)

1. _____ If your workplace has been able to institute many types of engineering controls, you don't need to use any personal protective equipment.

2. _____ According to the OSHA Bloodborne Pathogens Standard, ambulance services must install handwashing facilities in all ambulances.

3. _____ If an antiseptic hand cleanser or antiseptic towelette is used for handwashing, you must wash with soap and water as soon as possible.

4. _____ Drinking coffee is prohibited in work areas where there is a reasonable likelihood of occupational exposure to blood or OPIM.

B. Choose the best answer.

1. _____ Who is responsible for providing personal protective equipment to the employee, if the employee is or could be exposed to bloodborne pathogens at work?
   A. The employee
   B. The employer
   C. Both are partially responsible
   D. The customer

2. _____ Who is responsible for maintaining the personal protective equipment provided for the employee?
   A. The employee
   B. The employer
   C. Both are partially responsible
   D. The customer/client

3. _____ An example of a work practice control would be
   A. Latex gloves
   B. Puncture-resistant containers for used needles
   C. Handwashing to reduce contamination
   D. Face masks to reduce exposure

7

Housekeeping

■ **Work Surfaces** ■ **Sharps** ■
■ **Laundry** ■

Learning Objective

You will be able to explain how cleaning work surfaces and equipment will protect you from disease.

Work Surfaces

Your employer will identify which work surfaces could become contaminated with blood or OPIM. This could include, but is not limited to, wastebaskets, exam tables, counters, floors, ambulance interiors, and police cars.

A regular cleaning schedule will need to be established and followed. The schedule must consider location, type of surface, type of soil present, and procedure and tasks performed. The cleaning schedule must occur at least weekly or after completion of tasks, after contamination of surfaces, or at the end of a shift if there is a possibility of contamination.

While cleaning up potentially infectious materials, you will wear reusable latex gloves and use an EPA-approved solution. An example of an inexpensive approved solution is 10 percent bleach and water. You should use disposable towels to clean up the spill and then dispose of the towels in a biohazard-labeled bag. See Chapter 8.

Do not clean up broken glass with your hands. Instead use a dust pan and brush, cardboard, or tongs. Vacuum cleaners are prohibited for the cleaning of broken glass under the standard.

Broken glass must be placed in a sharps container. Placing broken glass in a plastic bag may put others at risk for an occupational exposure incident.

Sharps

Reusable sharps including pointed scissors that have been contaminated must be decontaminated before reuse. Before cleaning, store the sharps in a container with a wide opening and encourage people to use care in removing items.

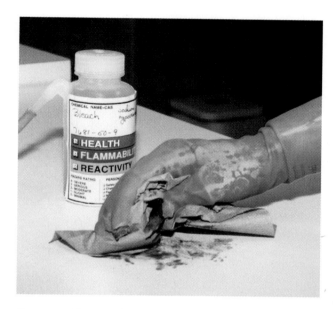

Care must be used when cleaning up contaminated spills.

Before decontamination, all visible blood or OPIM must be rinsed off, as large amounts of organic debris interfere with the efficacy of the disinfecting/sterilization process. *Never* blindly reach into any container.

Disposable sharps must be placed in puncture-resistant containers labeled as biohazardous to protect others. See Chapter 8.

Laundry

Laundry and waste materials may be separated into contaminated and noncontaminated labeled containers. Remember that the goal of these regulations is to protect you and others from contamination, so use plastic bags or double plastic bags (if the outside of the first bag becomes contaminated) to prevent leakage of wet/damp laundry.

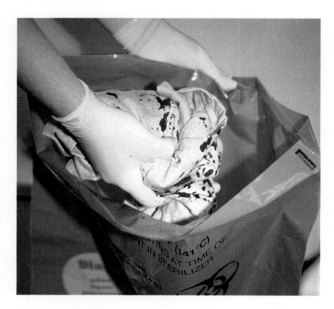

Contaminated laundry should be clearly labeled and placed in leakproof containers.

You must wear gloves when handling laundry or waste materials. Do not handle laundry any more than necessary. Home laundering of personal protective equipment is prohibited.

Contaminated laundry should be sent to a facility following the OSHA Standard.

■ HANDLING USED SHARPS ■

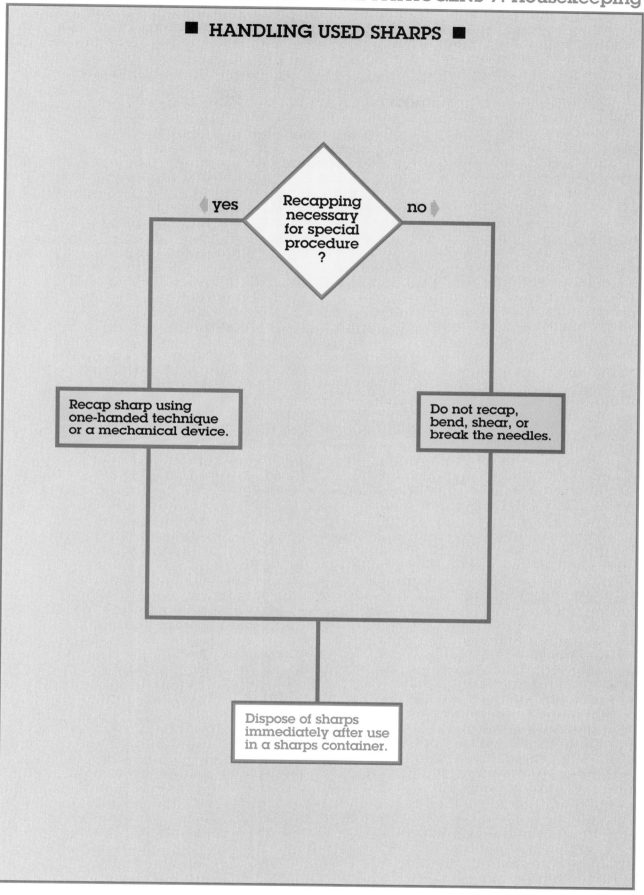

■ DISPOSAL OF SHARPS CONTAINERS ■

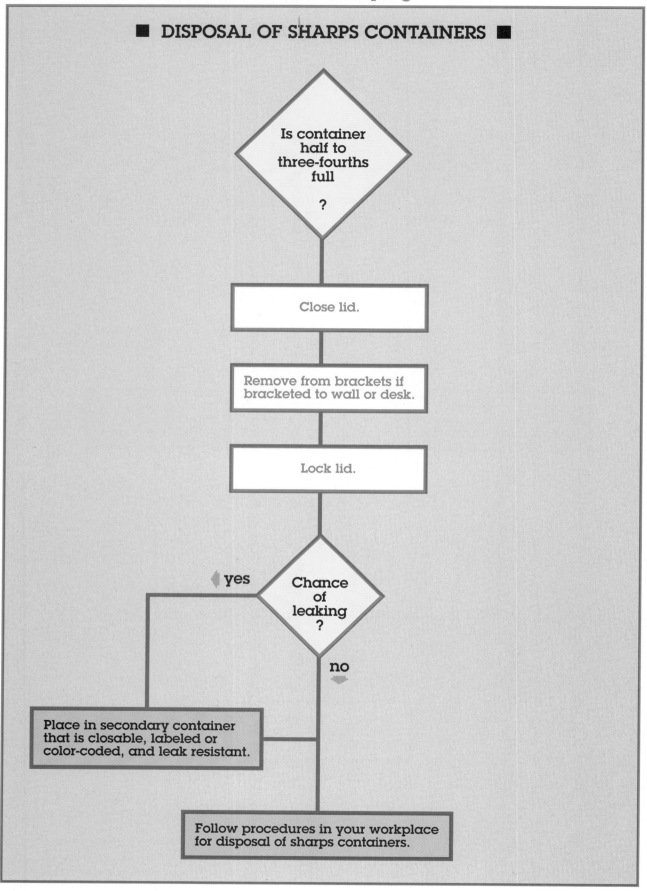

Is container half to three-fourths full ?

Close lid.

Remove from brackets if bracketed to wall or desk.

Lock lid.

Chance of leaking ?

yes

no

Place in secondary container that is closable, labeled or color-coded, and leak resistant.

Follow procedures in your workplace for disposal of sharps containers.

■ HANDLING CONTAMINATED LAUNDRY ■

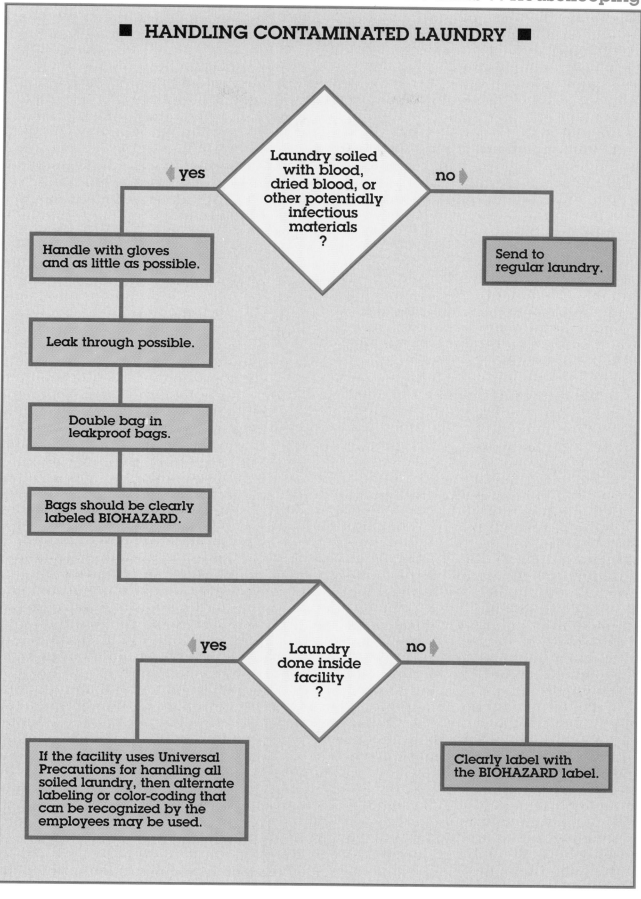

Laundry soiled with blood, dried blood, or other potentially infectious materials ?

yes → Handle with gloves and as little as possible.

no → Send to regular laundry.

Leak through possible.

Double bag in leakproof bags.

Bags should be clearly labeled BIOHAZARD.

Laundry done inside facility ?

yes → If the facility uses Universal Precautions for handling all soiled laundry, then alternate labeling or color-coding that can be recognized by the employees may be used.

no → Clearly label with the BIOHAZARD label.

Name _____ Course _____ Date _____

■ ACTIVITY 1 ■
Housekeeping

A. Mark each statement true (T) or false (F).

1. ____ While cleaning a spill of blood or other potentially infectious materials, gloves are not needed because of the cleaning solution used.

2. ____ A cleaning solution recommended to decontaminate a surface after a blood spill is a 10 percent bleach and water solution.

3. ____ Disposable sharps must be placed in some type of biohazard bag or container. The type of bag or container is unimportant as long as it says biohazard.

4. ____ Laundry does not need to be placed in a biohazard bag or labeled as biohazard because the OSHA standard does not apply to laundry.

5. ____ Persons handling regulated laundry, should practice Universal Precautions. This would include the wearing of latex gloves.

B. Choose the best answer.

1. ____ Which of the following would you *not* use to clean work surfaces.
    A. Disposable towels
    B. Reusable latex gloves
    C. Lysol and a wire brush
    D. 10 percent bleach and water solution

2. ____ If you have laundry with dried blood on it, you must
    A. Place it in a biohazard bag.
    B. Put it in a regular laundry bag because the blood is dried.
    C. Attach a label to that area of the laundry, thus letting people know that it is a biohazard.
    D. Soak the dried blood off in the nearest sink, and then place the laundry in the regular laundry bag.

8

Labeling

■ **What Is an Acceptable Container?** ■ **When Is Labeling Necessary?** ■
■ **Using Sharps Containers** ■ **Labeling Regulated Waste** ■

Learning Objective

You will be able to recognize and explain the appropriate labels and containers for containing contaminated items.

What Is an Acceptable Container?

A sharps container must meet four criteria to be considered acceptable.

It must be closable, puncture resistant, leakproof on sides and bottom, and labeled or color-coded.

A sharps container may be made of a variety of products including cardboard or plastic, as long as the four criteria are met. Duct tape may be used to secure a sharps container lid, but it is not acceptable if it serves as the lid itself.

When Is Labeling Necessary?

Labels must be provided on containers of regulated waste, on refrigerators and freezers that are used to store blood or OPIM, and on containers used to store, dispose of, transport, or ship blood or OPIM.

Equipment that is being sent to another facility for servicing or decontamination must have a label attached stating which portions of the equipment remain contaminated in order to warn other employees of the hazard and the precautions they need to take.

Using Sharps Containers

Contaminated sharps must be discarded immediately in an acceptable sharps container. Sharps containers must be easily accessible to personnel and located as close as feasible to the immediate area where sharps are used or can be reasonably anticipated to be found.

Sharps containers must be maintained upright throughout use and replaced routinely. The replace-

ment schedule must be clearly outlined in the Exposure Control Plan.

If leakage is possible, or if the outside of the container has become contaminated, the sharps container must be placed in a secondary container.

Areas such as correctional facilities, psychiatric units, or pediatric units may have difficulty placing sharps containers in the immediate use area. If a mobile cart is used by health care workers in these units, an alternative would be to lock a sharps container in the cart.

Laundries that handle contaminated laundry must have sharps containers easily accessible due to the incidence of needles mixed with laundry.

Facilities that handle shipments of waste that may contain contaminated sharps must also have sharps containers easily accessible in the event a package accidentally opens and releases sharps.

Labeling Regulated Waste

Regulated waste containers are required to be labeled with the biohazard label or color-coded to warn employees who may have contact with the containers of the potential hazard posed by their contents.

Even if your facility considers all of its waste to be regulated waste, the waste containers must still bear the required label or color-coding in order to protect new employees and employees from outside facilities.

Regulated waste that has been decontaminated need not be labeled or color-coded. However, your employer must have controls in place to determine if the decontamination process is successful.

Exceptions to Labeling Requirements

Blood and blood products that bear an identifying label as specified by the Food and Drug Administration and that have been screened for HBV and HIV antibodies and released for transfusion or other clinical uses are exempted from the labeling requirements.

When blood is being drawn or laboratory procedures are being performed on blood samples, then the individual containers housing the blood or OPIM do not have to be labeled provided the larger container into which they are placed for storage, transport, shipment, or disposal (for example, a test tube rack) is labeled.

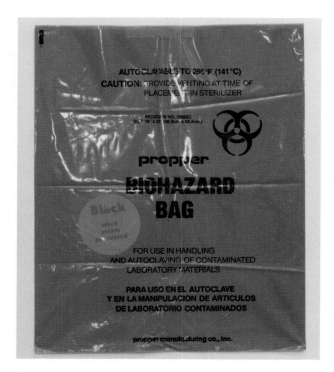

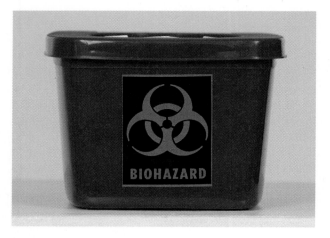

Biohazard symbols must be fluorescent orange or orange-red with letters or symbols in a contrasting color. These are attached to any container that is used to store or transport potentially infectious materials.

Biohazard labels may be attached to bags containing potentially infectious materials. The label must be fluorescent orange or orange-red in color and clearly visible.

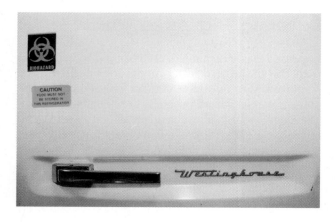

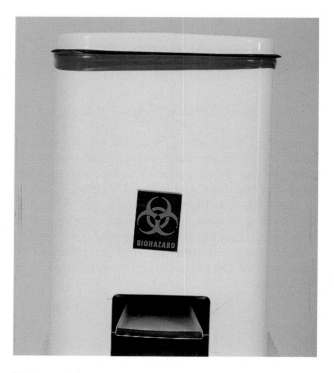

Biohazard labels must be fluorescent orange or orange-red in color and attached as close as feasible to the container by string, wire, adhesive, or other method that prevents their loss or unintentional removal.

Biohazard labels may be attached to waste containers containing potentially infectious materials. The label must be fluorescent orange or orange-red and clearly visible.

Name _____ Course _____ Date _____

■ ACTIVITY 1 ■
Labeling

A. Choose the best answer.

According to the OSHA Bloodborne Pathogen Standard, how must biohazardous substances be labeled?

A. _____ As long as they are clearly labeled it is satisfactory.

B. _____ The label must be fluorescent orange or orange-red in color with the biohazard symbol.

C. _____ Labeling is unnecessary if you are able to tell the person picking up the biohazardous material that it is biohazardous.

D. _____ The label must be fluorescent orange or orange-red with the biohazard symbol, and must be accompanied by a letter stating the type of material that is being handled.

B. Match the label or container with the activity.

A.
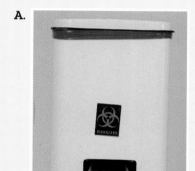

1. _____ You have just given an injection and need to dispose of the contaminated needle.

B.

2. _____ You have just cleaned up a spill in the lab and need to dispose of the paper towels.

C.

3. _____ You have just finished cleaning the ambulance and need to drop off the sheets used in transport.

9
Transmission

■ Mode of Transmission of Bloodborne Pathogens ■ Protecting Yourself ■
■ Handwashing ■ HBV versus HIV ■

Learning Objective

You will be able to explain how bloodborne pathogens are transmitted.

Mode of Transmission of Bloodborne Pathogens

Bloodborne pathogens are transmitted when blood or OPIM come in contact with mucous membranes, non-intact skin, or by handling or touching contaminated items or surfaces. Non-intact skin includes but is not limited to, cuts, abrasions, burns, rashes, paper cuts, and hangnails. Bloodborne pathogens are also trans-mitted by injection under the skin by puncture wounds or cuts from contaminated sharps.

The majority of occupational HIV transmission has occurred through puncture injury. However, there have been documented HIV transmissions from non-sexual, nonpercutaneous exposures to fresh blood or body fluid contamination with HIV. Transmission has been documented to occur after contact with HIV-contaminated blood through non-intact skin and mucous membranes. One worker became HIV positive after a splash of HIV contaminated blood to the eyes. It should be clear that contact with blood or OPIM should be avoided.

Protecting Yourself

To protect yourself from transmission of bloodborne pathogens, you should observe Universal Precautions and wear personal protective equipment.

Handwashing

Handwashing is one of the most effective methods of preventing transmission of bloodborne pathogens. It is required that you wash your hands after removal of gloves and other personal protective equipment.

HBV versus HIV

Hepatitis B Virus (HBV) is more persistent than HIV and is able to survive for at least a week in dried blood on environmental surfaces or contaminated instruments. It is unlikely that HIV will be transmitted by handling or touching contaminated surfaces whereas HBV is.

A source of HBV is chronic carriers. Chronic carriers have the antigen present at all times and can unwittingly transmit the disease to susceptible persons through transfusion, needle or other penetrating injury, and intimate contact.

A number of other bloodborne diseases other than HIV and HBV exist, such as Hepatitis C, Hepatitis D, and syphilis.

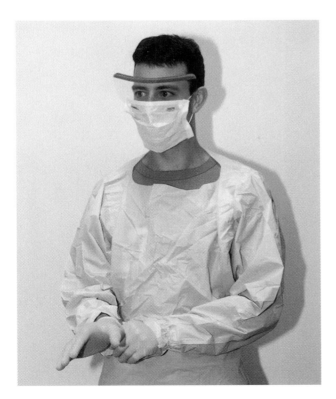

You can protect yourself from transmission of bloodborne pathogens.

Name _____ Course _____ Date _____

■ ACTIVITY 1 ■
Transmission

Mark each statement true (T) or false (F).

1. ____ Bloodborne pathogens are disease-causing microorganisms that can only be transmitted by direct contact with blood.

2. ____ Bloodborne pathogens may be transmitted through intact as well as non-intact skin.

3. ____ One of the most effective ways to prevent the spread of bloodborne pathogens is handwashing.

4. ____ HIV is considerably more persistent than HBV.

5. ____ HBV may be transmitted by handling or touching contaminated surfaces.

10
Exposure Determination

■ What Is an Occupational Exposure Incident? ■
■ Assessing Exposure Determination ■

Learning Objective

You will be able to determine whether an exposure incident could occur within your job.

What Is an Occupational Exposure Incident?

An occupational exposure incident occurs if you are in a work situation and come in contact with blood or other potentially infectious materials.

For OSHA 200 record-keeping purposes, an occupational bloodborne pathogens exposure incident (e.g., needlestick, laceration, or splash) shall be classified as an injury since it is usually the result of an instantaneous event or exposure.

Once an occupational exposure to blood or other potentially infectious materials has occurred, the employee's name and job classification are listed on the OSHA 200 log. All staff in the same job classification as the exposed employee are now covered under the standard and must receive the training and be offered the Hepatitis B immunization series at no cost.

Assessing Exposure Determination

Occupational exposure can occur in many different job situations. Examples of professions in which a person might be exposed to blood or OPIM could include, but are not limited to, physicians, nurses, police officers, ambulance attendants, EMTs, fire and rescue personnel, laboratory personnel, morticians and embalmers, and teachers. All persons in these professions need to be aware of their possible risk of exposure.

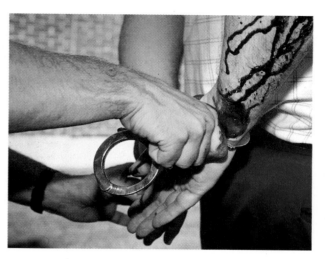

Are you at risk?

Any exposure is enough to place your job under the requirements of the standard. If you have ever been exposed to blood or OPIM, ask yourself why you have been exposed. Is the task that you were doing a normal part of your occupation? Was a package not properly labeled? Are you trained to prevent injury to yourself?

Name _____ Course _____ Date _____

■ ACTIVITY 1 ■
Exposure Risks

Put a check (✓) beside each example of possible job exposure.

1. _____ A nurse who is a teacher in a community college setting. At times, he does some hands-on nursing in the nearby hospital.

2. _____ The librarian at your local library who deals with all age groups.

3. _____ An embalmer at a funeral home in a large city.

4. _____ A dentist in any setting.

5. _____ The maintenance person who empties the trash at a hospital.

6. _____ Coach of a basketball team.

7. _____ Police officer subduing a violent prisoner.

8. _____ Lifeguard on duty at the local pool.

9. _____ Receptionist at a dental clinic.

■ ACTIVITY 2 ■
Risk Assessment

1. Do you have job exposure to blood or OPIM?

2. List three activities in your profession in which you could be exposed to blood or OPIM.

_____

_____

_____

_____

_____

_____

_____

3. What steps can you take to decrease your risk of an exposure incident involving bloodborne pathogens?

_____

_____

_____

_____

_____

_____

11
Post-Exposure Reporting

■ Minimizing Exposure ■ Reporting an Incident ■
■ Medical Care after an Incident ■ Confidentiality ■

Learning Objective

You will be able to describe the steps to take after an exposure incident and the importance of reporting it.

Minimizing Exposure

If you have an exposure incident to another person's blood or OPIM, immediately wash the exposed area with warm water and soap.

If the exposed area was in your mouth, rinse your mouth with water or mouthwash (whichever is most readily available).

If the exposure was in your eyes, flush with warm water (or normal saline if available). A quick rinse is probably not adequate, you want to irrigate the area completely with water.

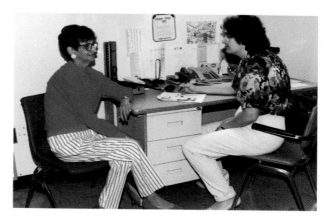

It is important to report all occupational exposure incidents immediately.

Reporting an Incident

Next report the incident to your supervisor. OSHA requires the following information:

1. How, when, and where the incident occurred.

2. With whose blood or body secretions did you come in contact? If you do not know, do not worry. Just explain why you do not know.

3. Your blood may be tested for HBV and/or HIV only with your consent. You may refuse. But you may also have the blood drawn and stored for 90 days. If you change your mind within the 90 days, HIV testing will be done. If you elect not to have the blood tested, the sample will be disposed of without testing after 90 days.

4. The source individual's blood will also be tested if available (unless already known to be HIV or HBV positive) and the results of the test will be made known to you. State laws may vary, please check with your instructor regarding confidentiality laws in your state.

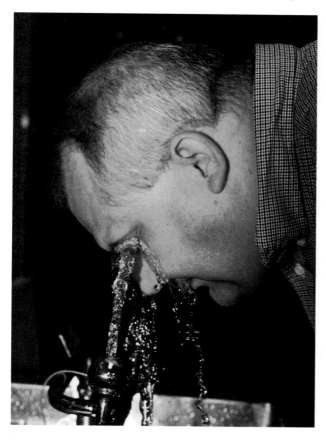

To minimize exposure, flush affected area immediately with water.

Medical Care after an Incident

You are entitled to medical care after an exposure incident. When you go for treatment the following information will be made available to the caregiver.

1. A copy of the OSHA guidelines section 1910.1030

2. A description of how the incident occurred as it relates to your employment

3. The results of the source individual's testing (if available)

4. All medical records that pertain to this one incident

The following is a list of the records that your employer is required to have on file about each employee:

1. The name and social security number of each employee

2. A copy of the employee's Hepatitis B vaccination status including the dates of all the Hepatitis B vaccinations and any medical records relative to the employee's ability to receive the vaccination

3. A copy of all results of examinations, medical testing, and follow-up procedures after an exposure incident

4. The employer's copy of the health care provider's written opinion regarding the incident

Confidentiality

It is the employer's responsibility to ensure that employee medical records are kept confidential. Your records cannot be disclosed without your express written consent to any person within or outside the workplace except as required by law.

Name _____ Course _____ Date _____

■ ACTIVITY 1 ■
Post-Exposure Reporting

A. After reading the following scenario, check (✓) the steps that you should take.

You have had a long day in the lab and your final patient is a 2-year-old child. You have successfully drawn the needed blood and are transferring the blood to a glass container. The child accidentally strikes the container, the container smashes to the floor, and the needle pierces through your glove into your hand. At this point you should:

1. ____ Clean up the glass shards with your hands.

2. ____ Report the incident to your supervisor.

3. ____ Decontaminate the area with a 10 percent bleach and water solution.

4. ____ Put on reusable latex gloves.

5. ____ Dispose of the shards of glass in the trash.

6. ____ Use paper towels to soak up most of the spill.

7. ____ Dispose of the blood-soaked paper towels in a sharps container.

8. ____ Wash you hands thoroughly with soap and warm water.

B. Check (✓) the post-exposure items that should occur and to which you are entitled following exposure to blood or potentially infectious material.

1. ____ Report how, when, and where the incident occurred.

2. ____ Report whose blood or body secretions you came in contact with.

3. ____ You must know where the blood or body secretions came from.

4. ____ You may have your blood tested for HIV and/or HBV immediately.

5. ____ If your blood is not tested immediately, it may not be tested later.

6. ____ If your blood is drawn but not tested immediately, it may be tested up to 90 days later.

7. ____ The source individual's blood must be tested, but you will not know the results.

12
Requirements
■ The Exposure Control Plan ■

Learning Objective

You will be able to state the requirements of the Exposure Control Plan.

The Exposure Control Plan

Each employer having an employee with occupational exposure to blood or OPIM shall establish a written Exposure Control Plan designed to eliminate or minimize employee exposure.

The Exposure Control Plan shall contain at least:

1. An exposure determination including:

   a. A list of job classifications in which occupational exposure may occur, and will occur

   b. A list of all tasks and procedures in which occupational exposure occurs and that are performed by employees in the job classifications listed above

2. This Exposure Control Plan shall be written as if personal protective equipment is not used. Personal protective equipment should be used as a back up method only, not primary protection.

3. The schedule and method of implementation of methods of compliance including:

   a. Universal Precautions

   b. Engineering Controls

   c. Work practice controls

   d. Hepatitis B vaccination and post-exposure evaluation and follow-up

   e. Communication and record keeping procedures

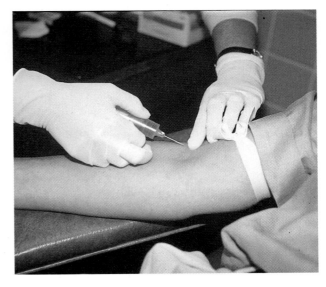

All procedures that risk occupational exposure are outlined in the Exposure Control Plan.

4. Each employer shall ensure that a copy of the Exposure Control Plan is accessible to employees in accordance with 29 CFR 1910.30 (the OSHA Bloodborne Pathogen Standard).

5. The Exposure Control Plan shall be renewed and updated annually and whenever necessary to reflect new or modified tasks and procedures that affect occupational exposure, and to reflect new or revised employee positions with occupational exposure.

6. The Exposure Control Plan shall be made available to the Assistant Secretary of Labor and the Director on request.

Name _____ Course _____ Date _____

■ ACTIVITY 1 ■
The Exposure Control Plan

Choose the best answer.

1. ____ The Exposure Control Plan does not need to include:
   A. A schedule and method of implementation
   B. A list of job classifications and exposure risks
   C. The names of all employees
   D. A copy of the plan available to all employees

2. ____ The Exposure Control Plan must be updated:
   A. Monthly
   B. Annually
   C. Whenever the regulations are changed
   D. Both B and C

3. ____ The responsibility to develop the Exposure Control Plan belongs to
   A. The employee in that department
   B. The employer
   C. OSHA
   D. The employees who are at risk for exposure incidents

Appendix A
Glossary

A

AFB: Acid-fast bacilli.

AIDS: Acquired Immunodeficiency Syndrome, a disease that results from HIV.

airborne: Capable of being transmitted by air particles.

anorexia: Loss of appetite.

antigen: A substance that causes antibody formation.

B

blood: The OSHA Standard refers to human blood, human blood components, and products made with human blood.

bloodborne pathogen: A pathogenic microorganism that is present in human blood and can cause disease in humans.

C

contaminated: The presence or the reasonably anticipated presence of blood or other potentially infectious materials on an item or surface.

contaminated laundry: Laundry that has been soiled with blood or other potentially infectious materials or may contain sharps.

contaminated sharps: Any contaminated object that can penetrate the skin including, but not limited to, needles, scalpels, broken capillary tubes, and exposed ends of dental wires.

D

decontamination: The use of physical or chemical means to remove, inactivate, or destroy bloodborne pathogens on a surface or item to the point where they are no longer capable of transmitting infectious particles and the surface or item is rendered safe for handling, use, or disposal.

DeLee suctioning: An emergency method of clearing an infant's airway.

E

engineering controls: Physical controls (e.g., sharps disposal containers, self-sheathing needles, etc.) that isolate or remove the bloodborne pathogens hazard from the workplace.

exposure incident: A specific eye, mouth, other mucous membrane, non-intact skin, or parenteral contact with blood or other potentially infectious materials that results from the performance of an employee's duties.

extrapulmonary: Outside of the lungs.

H

handwashing facility: A facility that provides an adequate supply of running potable water, soap, and single use towels or hot air drying machines.

HBV: Hepatitis B Virus. One of the viruses that causes illness directly affecting the liver. It is a bloodborne pathogen.

HEPA: High-efficiency particulate air filter.

hepatitis: A disease that causes swelling, soreness, and loss of normal function of the liver. Symptoms include weakness, fatigue, anorexia, nausea, abdominal pain, fever, and headache. Jaundice is a symptom that may develop later.

HIV: Human Immunodeficiency Virus is a virus that infects immune system blood cells in humans and renders them less effective in preventing disease.

I

immune: Resistant to infectious disease.

immunization: A process or procedure by which resistance to infectious disease is produced in a person.

J

jaundice: A yellowing of the skin associated with hepatitis infection.

M

mucous membrane: Any one of the four types of thin sheets of tissue that cover or line various parts of the body. An example would be the skin lining the nose and mouth.

mucus: The clear secretion of the mucous membrane.

N

non-intact skin: Skin that has a break in the surface. It includes but is not limited to abrasions, cuts, hangnails, paper cuts, and burns.

nuclei: A particle that makes up a nucleus of an atom.

O

occupational: Job related.

occupational exposure: Reasonably anticipated skin, eye, mucous membrane, or parenteral contact with blood or other potentially infectious materials that may result from the performance of an employee's duties.

P

parenteral: Piercing mucous membranes or the skin barrier through such events as needle sticks, human bites, cuts, and abrasion.

pathogen: Any virus, microorganism, or other substance that is capable of causing disease.

percutaneous: Performed through the skin as in draining fluid from an abscess using a needle.

personal protective equipment: Specialized clothing or equipment worn by an employee for protection against hazard.

R

respirator: A mechanical device used to assist breathing. In this case it refers to a device used to filter particles from the air.

S

source individual: Any individual, living or dead, whose blood or other potentially infectious materials may be a source of occupational exposure to the employee.

sterilize: The use of a physical or chemical procedure to destroy all microbial life.

T

T$_4$: A cell in the immune system that acts as a sensor to activate the immune system.

TB disease: Having the organism that causes TB in the body, in its active state. A person with TB disease usually has symptoms and can transmit the disease to others.

TB infection: Having the organism that causes TB in the body, but not having the active disease. A person having TB infection is asymptomatic and cannot transmit TB unless the organism converts to an active state.

U

Universal Precautions: A comprehensive approach to infection control that treats all human blood and certain human body fluids as if known to be infectious for HIV, HBV, and other bloodborne pathogens.

V

vaccine: A suspension of inactive or killed microorganisms administered orally or injected into a human to induce active immunity to infectious disease.

Appendix B
OSHA Bloodborne Pathogens Standard

OSHA Bloodborne Pathogens Regulations Section 1910.1030

Part 1910-[Amended]

Subpart Z-[Amended]

1. The general authority citation for subpart Z of 29 CFR part 1910 continues to read as follows and a new citation for 1910.1030 is added:

Authority: Secs. 6 and 8, Occupational Safety and Health Act, 29 U.S.C. 655, 657, Secretary of Labor's Orders Nos. 12-71 (36 CFR 8754), 8-76 (41 CFR 25059), or 9-83 (48 CFR 35736), as applicable; and 29 CFR part 1911.

*   *   *

Section 1910.1030 also issued under 29 U.S.C. 853.

*   *   *

2. Section 1910.1030 is added to read as follows:

1910.1030 Bloodborne Pathogens.

(a) Scope and Application

This section applies to all occupational exposure to blood or other potentially infectious materials as defined by paragraph (b) of this section.

(b) Definitions

For purposes of this section, the following shall apply:

Assistant Secretary means the Assistant Secretary of Labor for Occupational Safety and Health, or designated representative.

Blood means human blood, human blood components, and products made from human blood.

Bloodborne Pathogens means pathogenic microorganisms that are present in human blood and can cause disease in humans. These pathogens include, but are not limited to, Hepatitis B Virus [HBV] and Human Immunodeficiency Virus [HIV].

Clinical Laboratory means a workplace where diagnostic or other screening procedures are performed on blood or other potentially infectious materials.

Contaminated means the presence or the reasonably anticipated presence of blood or other potentially infectious materials on an item or surface.

Contaminated Laundry means laundry which has been soiled with blood or other potentially infectious materials or may contain sharps.

Contaminated Sharps means any contaminated object that can penetrate the skin including, but not limited to, needles, scalpels, broken glass, broken capillary tubes, and exposed ends of dental wires.

Decontamination means the use of physical or chemical means to remove, inactivate, or destroy bloodborne pathogens on a surface or item to the point where they are no longer capable of transmitting infectious particles and the surface or item is rendered safe for handling, use, or disposal.

Director means the Director of the National Institute for Occupational Safety and Health, U.S. Department of Health and Human Services, or designated representative.

Engineering Controls means controls (e.g., sharps disposal containers, self-sheathing needles) that isolate or remove the bloodborne pathogens hazard from the workplace.

Exposure Incident means a specific eye, mouth, other mucous membrane, non-intact skin, or parenteral contact with blood or other potentially infectious materials that results from the performance of an employee's duties.

Handwashing Facilities means a facility providing an adequate supply of running potable water, soap, and single use towels or hot air drying machines.

Licensed Health Care Professional is a person whose legally permitted scope of practice allows him or her to independently perform the activities required by paragraph (f) Hepatitis B vaccination and Post-Exposure Evaluation and Follow-Up.

HBV means Hepatitis B Virus.

HIV means Human Immunodeficiency Virus.

Occupational Exposure means reasonably anticipated skin, eye, mucous membrane, or parenteral contact with blood or other potentially infectious materials that may result from the performance of an employee's duties.

Other Potentially Infectious Materials means

(1) The following human body fluids: semen, vaginal secretions, cerebrospinal fluid, synovial fluid, pleural fluid, pericardial fluid, peritoneal fluid, amniotic fluid, saliva in dental procedures, any body fluid that is visibly contaminated with blood, and all body fluids in situations where it is difficult or impossible to differentiate between body fluids;

(2) Any unfixed tissue or organ (other than intact skin) from a human (living or dead); and

(3) HIV-containing cell or tissue cultures, organ cultures, and HIV- or HBV-containing culture medium or other solutions; and blood, organs, or other tissues from experimental animals infected with HIV or HBV.

Parenteral means piercing mucous membranes or the skin barrier through such events as needlesticks, human bites, cuts, and abrasions.

Personal Protective Equipment is specialized clothing or equipment worn by an employee for protection against a hazard. General work clothes (e.g., uniforms, pants, shirts, or blouses) not intended to function as protection against a hazard are not considered to be personal protective equipment.

Production Facility means a facility engaged in industrial-scale, large-volume, or high concentration production of HIV or HBV.

Regulated Waste means liquid or semi-liquid blood or other potentially infectious materials; contaminated items that would release blood or other potentially infectious materials in a liquid or semi-liquid state if compressed; items that are caked with dried blood or other potentially infectious materials and are capable of releasing these materials during handling; contaminated sharps; and pathological and microbiological wastes containing blood or other potentially infectious materials.

Research Laboratory means a laboratory producing or using research-laboratory-scale amounts of HIV or HBV. Research laboratories may produce high concentrations of HIV or HBV but not in the volume found in production facilities.

Source Individual means any individual, living or dead, whose blood or other potentially infectious materials may be a source of occupational exposure to the employee. Examples include, but are not limited to, hospital and clinic patients; clients in institutions for the developmentally disabled; trauma victims; clients of drug and alcohol treatment facilities; residents of hospices and nursing homes; human remains; and individuals who donate or sell blood or blood components.

Sterilize means the use of a physical or chemical procedure to destroy all microbial life including highly resistant bacterial endospores.

Universal Precautions is an approach to infection control. According to the concept of Universal Precautions, all human blood and certain human body fluids are treated as if known to be infectious for HIV, HBV, and other blood-borne pathogens.

Work Practice Controls means controls that reduce the likelihood of exposure by altering the manner in which a task is performed (e.g., prohibiting recapping of needles by a two-handed technique).

(c) Exposure Control

(1) *Exposure Control Plan.*

(i) Each employer having an employee(s) with occupational exposure as defined by paragraph (b) of this section shall establish a written Exposure Control Plan designed to eliminate or minimize employee exposure.

(ii) The Exposure Control Plan shall contain at least the following elements:

(A) The exposure determination required by paragraph (c)(2);

(B) The schedule and method of implementation for paragraphs (d) Methods of Compliance, (e) HIV and HBV Research Laboratories and Production Facilities, (f) Hepatitis B Vaccination and Post-Exposure Evaluation and Follow-Up, (g) Communication of Hazards to Employees, and (h) Recordkeeping of this standard; and

(C) The procedure for the evaluation of circumstances surrounding exposure incidents as required by paragraph (f)(3)(i) of this standard.

(iii) Each employer shall ensure that a copy of the Exposure Control Plan is accessible to employees in accordance with 29 CFR 1910.20(e).

(iv) The Exposure Control Plan shall be reviewed and updated at least annually and whenever necessary to reflect new or modified tasks and procedures which affect occupational exposure and to reflect new or revised employee positions with occupational exposure.

(v) The Exposure Control Plan shall be made available to the Assistant Secretary and the Director upon request for examination and copying.

(2) *Exposure Determination.*

(i) Each employer who has an employee(s) with occupational exposure as defined by paragraph (b) of this section shall prepare an exposure determination. This exposure determination shall contain the following:

(A) A list of all job classifications in which all employees in those job classifications have occupational exposure;

(B) A list of job classifications in which some employees have occupational exposure; and

(C) A list of all tasks and procedures or groups of closely related task and procedures in which occupational exposures occur and that are performed by employees in job classifications listed in accordance with the provisions of paragraph (c)(2)(i)(B) of this standard.

(ii) This exposure determination shall be made without regard to the use of personal protective equipment.

(d) Methods of Compliance

(1) *General.*

Universal precautions shall be observed to prevent contact with blood or other potentially infectious materials. Under circumstances in which differentiation between body fluid types is difficult or impossible, all body fluids shall be considered potentially infectious materials.

(2) *Engineering and Work Practice Controls.*

(i) Engineering and work practice controls shall be used to eliminate or minimize employee exposure. Where occupational exposure remains after institution of these controls, personal protective equipment shall also be used.

(ii) Engineering controls shall be examined and maintained or replaced on a regular schedule to ensure their effectiveness.

(iii) Employers shall provide handwashing facilities which are readily accessible to employees.

(iv) When provision of handwashing facilities is not feasible, the employer shall provide either an appropriate antiseptic hand cleanser in conjunction with clean cloth/paper towels or antiseptic towelettes. When antiseptic hand cleansers or towelettes are used, hands shall be washed with soap and running water as soon as feasible.

(v) Employers shall ensure that employees wash their hands immediately or as soon as feasible after removal of gloves or other personal protective equipment.

(vi) Employers shall ensure that employees wash hands and any other skin with soap and water, or flush mucous membranes with water immediately or as soon as feasible following contact of such body areas with blood or other potentially infectious materials.

(vii) Contaminated needles and other contaminated sharps shall not be bent, recapped, or removed except as noted in paragraphs (d)(2)(vii)(A) and (d)(2)(vii)(B) below. Shearing or breaking of contaminated needles is prohibited.

  (A) Contaminated needles and other contaminated sharps shall not be recapped or removed unless the employer can demonstrate that no alternative is feasible or that such action is required by a specific medical procedure.

  (B) Such recapping or needle removal must be accomplished through the use of a mechanical device or a one-handed technique.

(viii) Immediately or as soon as possible after use, contaminated reusable sharps shall be placed in appropriate containers until properly reprocessed. These containers shall be:

  (A) Puncture resistant;

  (B) Labeled or color-coded in accordance with this standard;

  (C) Leakproof on the sides and bottom; and

  (D) In accordance with the requirements set forth in paragraph (d)(4)(ii)(E) for reusable sharps.

(ix) Eating, drinking, smoking, applying cosmetics or lip balm, and handling contact lenses are prohibited in work areas where there is a reasonable likelihood of occupational exposure.

(x) Food and drink shall not be kept in refrigerators, freezers, shelves, cabinets or on countertops or benchtops where blood or other potentially infectious materials are present.

(xi) All procedures involving blood or other potentially infectious materials shall be performed in such a manner as to minimize splashing, spraying, spattering, and generation of droplets of these substances.

(xii) Mouth pipetting/suctioning of blood or other potentially infectious materials is prohibited.

(xiii) Specimens of blood or other potentially infectious materials shall be placed in a container which prevents leakage during collection, handling, processing, storage, transport, or shipping.

  (A) The container for storage, transport, or shipping shall be labeled or color-coded according to paragraph (g)(1)(i) and closed prior to being stored, transported, or shipped. When a facility utilizes Universal Precautions in the handling of all specimens, the labeling/color-coding of specimens is not necessary provided containers are recognizable as containing specimens. This exemption only applies while such specimens/containers remain within the facility. Labeling or color-coding in accordance with paragraph (g)(1)(i) is required when such specimens/containers leave the facility.

  (B) If outside contamination of the primary container occurs, the primary container shall be placed within a second container which prevents leakage during handling, processing, storage, transport, or shipping and is labeled or color-coded according to the requirements of this standard.

  (C) If the specimen could puncture the primary container, the primary container shall be placed within a secondary container which is puncture-resistant in addition to the above characteristics.

(xiv) Equipment which may become contaminated with blood or other potentially infectious materials shall be examined prior to servicing or shipping and shall be decontaminated as necessary, unless the employer can demonstrate that decontamination of such equipment or portions of such equipment is not feasible.

  (A) A readily observable label in accordance with paragraph (g)(1)(i)(H) shall be attached to the equipment stating which portions remain contaminated.

  (B) The employer shall ensure that this information is conveyed to all affected employees, the servicing representative, and/or the manufacturer, as appropriate, prior to handling, servicing, or shipping so that appropriate precautions will be taken.

(3) *Personal Protective Equipment.*

  (i) Provision. When there is occupational exposure, the employer shall provide, at no cost to the employee, appropriate personal protective equipment such as, but not limited to, gloves, gowns, laboratory coats, face shields or masks and eye protection, and mouthpieces, resuscitation bags, pocket masks, or other ventilation devices. Personal protective equipment will be considered "appropriate" only if it does not permit blood or other potentially infectious materials to pass through to or reach the employee's work clothes, street clothes, undergarments, skin, eyes, mouth, or other mucous membranes under normal conditions of use and for the duration of time which the protective equipment will be used.

(ii) Use. The employer shall ensure that the employee uses appropriate personal protective equipment unless the employer shows that the employee temporarily and briefly declined to use personal protective equipment when, under rare and extraordinary circumstances, it was the employee's professional judgment that in the specific instance its use would have prevented the delivery of health care or public safety services or would have posed an increased hazard to the safety of the worker or co-worker. When the employee makes this judgment, the circumstances shall be investigated and documented in order to determine whether changes can be instituted to prevent such occurrences in the future.

(iii) Accessibility. The employer shall ensure that appropriate personal protective equipment in the appropriate sizes is readily accessible at the worksite or is issued to employees. Hypoallergenic gloves, glove liners, powderless gloves, or other similar alternatives shall be readily accessible to those employees who are allergic to the gloves normally provided.

(iv) Cleaning, Laundering, and Disposal. The employer shall clean, launder, and dispose of personal protective equipment required by paragraphs (d) and (e) of this standard, at no cost to the employee.

(v) Repair and Replacement. The employer shall repair or replace personal protective equipment as needed to maintain its effectiveness, at no cost to the employee.

(vi) If a garment(s) is penetrated by blood or other potentially infectious materials, the garment(s) shall be removed immediately or as soon as feasible.

(vii) All personal protective equipment shall be removed prior to leaving the work area.

(viii) When personal protective equipment is removed it shall be placed in an appropriately designated area or container for storage, washing, decontamination, or disposal.

(ix) Gloves. Gloves shall be worn when it can be reasonably anticipated that the employee may have hand contact with blood, other potentially infectious materials, mucous membranes, and non-intact skin; when performing vascular access procedures except as specified in paragraph (d)(3)(ix)(D); and when handling or touching contaminated items or surfaces.

(A) Disposable (single-use) gloves such as surgical or examination gloves, shall be replaced as soon as practical when contaminated or as soon as feasible if they are torn, punctured, or when their ability to function as a barrier is compromised.

(B) Disposable (single-use) gloves shall not be washed or decontaminated for re-use.

(C) Utility gloves may be decontaminated for reuse if the integrity of the glove is not compromised. However, they must be discarded if they are cracked, peeling, torn, punctured, or exhibit other signs of deterioration or when their ability to function as a barrier is compromised.

(D) If an employer in a volunteer blood donation center judges that routine gloving for all phlebotomies is not necessary then the employer shall:

(1) Periodically reevaluate this policy;

(2) Make gloves available to all employees who wish to use them for phlebotomy;

(3) Not discourage the use of gloves for phlebotomy; and

(4) Require that gloves be used for phlebotomy in the following circumstances:

(i) When the employee has cuts, scratches, or other breaks in his or her skin;

(ii) When the employee judges that hand contamination with blood may occur, for example, when performing phlebotomy on an uncooperative source individual; and

(iii) When the employee is receiving training in phlebotomy.

(x) Masks, Eye Protection, and Face Shields. Masks in combination with eye protection devices, such as goggles or glasses with solid side shields, or chin-length face shields, shall be worn whenever splashes, spray, spatter, or droplets of blood or other potentially infectious materials may be generated and eye, nose, or mouth contamination can be reasonably anticipated.

(xi) Gowns, Aprons, and Other Protective Body Clothing. Appropriate protective clothing such as, but not limited to, gowns, aprons, lab coats, clinic jackets, or similar outer garments shall be worn in occupational exposure situations. The type and characteristics will depend upon the task and degree of exposure anticipated.

(xii) Surgical caps or hoods and/or shoe covers or boots shall be worn in instances when gross contamination can reasonably be anticipated (e.g., autopsies, orthopedic surgery).

(4) *Housekeeping.*

(i) General. Employers shall ensure that the worksite is maintained in a clean and sanitary condition. The employer shall determine and implement an appropriate written schedule for cleaning and method of decontamination based upon the location within the facility, type of surface to be cleaned, type of soil present, and tasks or procedures being performed in the area.

(ii) All equipment and environmental and working surfaces shall be cleaned and decontaminated after contact with blood or other potentially infectious materials.

(A) Contaminated work surfaces shall be decontaminated with an appropriate disinfectant after completion of procedures; immediately or as soon as feasible when surfaces are overtly contaminated or after any spill of blood or other potentially infectious materials; and at the end of the work shift if the surface may have become contaminated since the last cleaning.

(B) Protective coverings, such as plastic wrap, aluminum foil, or imperviously backed absorbent paper used to cover equipment and environmental surfaces, shall be removed and replaced as soon as feasible when they become overtly contaminated or at the end of the work shift if they may have become contaminated during the shift.

(C) All bins, pails, cans, and similar receptacles intended for reuse which have a reasonable likelihood for becoming contaminated with blood or other potentially infectious materials shall be inspected and decontaminated on a regularly scheduled basis and cleaned and decontaminated immediately or as soon as feasible upon visible contamination.

(D) Broken glassware which may be contaminated shall not be picked up directly with the hands. It shall be cleaned up using mechanical means, such as a brush and dust pan, tongs, or forceps.

(E) Reusable sharps that are contaminated with blood or other potentially infectious materials shall not be stored or processed in a manner that requires employees to reach by hand into the containers where these sharps have been placed.

(iii) Regulated Waste.

(A) Contaminated Sharps Discarding and Containment.

(1) Contaminated sharps shall be discarded immediately or as soon as feasible in containers that are:

(i) Closable;

(ii) Puncture resistant;

(iii) Leakproof on sides and bottom; and

(iv) Labeled or color-coded in accordance with paragraph (g)(1)(i) of this standard.

(2) During use, containers for contaminated sharps shall be:

(i) Easily accessible to personnel and located as close as is feasible to the immediate area where sharps are used or can be reasonably anticipated to be found (e.g., laundries);

(ii) Maintained upright throughout use; and

(iii) Replaced routinely and not be allowed to overfill.

(3) When moving containers of contaminated sharps from the area of use, the containers shall be:

(i) Closed immediately prior to removal or replacement to prevent spillage or protrusion of contents during handling, storage, transport, or shipping;

(ii) Placed in a secondary container if leakage is possible. The second container shall be:

(A) Closable;

(B) Constructed to contain all contents and prevent leakage during handling, storage, transport, or shipping; and

(C) Labeled or color-coded according to paragraph (g)(1)(i) of this standard.

(4) Reusable containers shall not be opened, emptied, or cleaned manually or in any other manner which would expose employees to the risk of percutaneous injury.

(B) Regulated Waste Containment.

(1) Regulated waste shall be placed in containers that are:

(i) Closable;

(ii) Constructed to contain all contents and prevent leakage of fluids during handling, storage, transport, or shipping;

(iii) Labeled or color-coded in accordance with paragraph (g)(1)(i) of this standard; and

(iv) Closed prior to removal to prevent spillage or protrusion of contents during handling, storage, transport, or shipping.

(2) If outside contamination of the regulated waste container occurs, it shall be placed in a second container. The second container shall be:

(i) Closable;

(ii) Constructed to contain all contents and prevent leakage of fluids during handling, storage, transport, or shipping;

(iii) Labeled or color-coded in accordance with paragraph (g)(1)(i) of this standard; and

(iv) Closed prior to removal to prevent spillage or protrusion of contents during handling, storage, transport, or shipping.

(C) Disposal of all regulated waste shall be in accordance with applicable regulations of the United States, States and Territories, and political subdivisions of States and Territories.

(iv) Laundry.

   (A) Contaminated laundry shall be handled as little as possible with a minimum of agitation.

   (1) Contaminated laundry shall be bagged or containerized at the location where it was used and shall not be sorted or rinsed in the location of use.

   (2) Contaminated laundry shall be placed and transported in bags or containers labeled or color-coded in accordance with paragraph (g)(1)(i) of this standard. When a facility utilizes Universal Precautions in the handling of all soiled laundry, alternative labeling or color-coding is sufficient if it permits all employees to recognize the containers as requiring compliance with Universal Precautions.

   (3) Whenever contaminated laundry is wet and presents a reasonable likelihood of soak-through of or leakage from the bag or container, the laundry shall be placed and transported in bags or containers which prevent soak-through and/or leakage of fluids to the exterior.

   (B) The employer shall ensure that employees who have contact with contaminated laundry wear protective gloves and other appropriate personal protective equipment.

   (C) When a facility ships contaminated laundry off-site to a second facility which does not utilize Universal Precautions in the handling of all laundry, the facility generating the contaminated laundry must place such laundry in bags or containers which are labeled or color-coded in accordance with paragraph (g)(1)(i).

(e) **HIV and HBV Research Laboratories and Production Facilities.**

   (1) This paragraph applies to research laboratories and production facilities engaged in the culture, production, concentration, experimentation, and manipulation of HIV and HBV. It does not apply to clinical or diagnostic laboratories engaged solely in the analysis of blood, tissues, or organs. These requirements apply in addition to the other requirements of the standard.

   (2) Research laboratories and production facilities shall meet the following criteria:

   (i) Standard microbiological practices. All regulated waste shall either be incinerated or decontaminated by a method such as autoclaving known to effectively destroy bloodborne pathogens.

   (ii) Special practices:

   (A) Laboratory doors shall be kept closed when work involving HIV or HBV is in progress.

   (B) Contaminated materials that are to be decontaminated at a site away from the work area shall be placed in a durable, leakproof, labeled or color-coded container that is closed before being removed from the work area.

   (C) Access to the work area shall be limited to authorized persons. Written policies and procedures shall be established whereby only persons who have been advised of the potential biohazard, who meet any specific entry requirements, and who comply with all entry and exit procedures shall be allowed to enter the work areas and animal rooms.

   (D) When other potentially infectious materials or infected animals are present in the work area or containment module, a hazard warning sign incorporating the universal biohazard symbol shall be posted on all access doors. The hazard warning sign shall comply with paragraph (g)(1)(ii) of this standard.

   (E) All activities involving other potentially infectious materials shall be conducted in biological safety cabinets or other physical-containment devices within the containment module. No work with these other potentially infectious materials shall be conducted on the open bench.

   (F) Laboratory coats, gowns, smocks, uniforms, or other appropriate protective clothing shall be used in the work area and animal rooms. Protective clothing shall not be worn outside of the work area and shall be decontaminated before being laundered.

   (G) Special care shall be taken to avoid skin contact with other potentially infectious materials. Gloves shall be worn when handling infected animals and when making hand contact with other potentially infectious materials is unavoidable.

   (H) Before disposal all waste from work areas and from animal rooms shall either be incinerated or decontaminated by a method such as autoclaving known to effectively destroy bloodborne pathogens.

   (I) Vacuum lines shall be protected with liquid disinfectant traps and high efficiency particulate air (HEPA) filters or filters of equivalent or superior efficiency and which are checked routinely and maintained or replaced as necessary.

   (J) Hypodermic needles and syringes shall be used only for parenteral injection and aspiration of fluids from laboratory animals and diaphragm bottles. Only needle-locking syringes or disposable syringe-needle units (i.e., the needle is integral to the syringe) shall be used for the injection or aspiration of other potentially infectious materials. Extreme caution shall be used when handling needles and syringes. A needle shall not be bent, sheared, replaced in the sheath or guard, or removed from the syringe following use. The needle and syringe shall be promptly placed in a puncture-resistant container and autoclaved or decontaminated before reuse or disposal.

(K) All spills shall be immediately contained and cleaned up by appropriate professional staff or others properly trained and equipped to work with potentially concentrated infectious materials.

(L) A spill or accident that results in an exposure incident shall be immediately reported to the laboratory director or other responsible person.

(M) A biosafety manual shall be prepared or adopted and periodically reviewed and updated at least annually or more often if necessary. Personnel shall be advised of potential hazards, shall be required to read instructions on practices and procedures, and shall be required to follow them.

(iii) Containment Equipment

(A) Certified biological safety cabinets (Class II, III, or IV) or other appropriate combinations of personal protection or physical containment devices, such as special protective clothing, respirators, centrifuge safety cups, sealed centrifuge rotors, and containment caging for animals, shall be used for all activities with other potentially infectious materials that pose a threat of exposure to droplets, splashes, spills, or aerosols.

(B) Biological safety cabinets shall be certified when installed, whenever they are moved, and at least annually.

(3) HIV and HBV research laboratories shall meet the following criteria:

(i) Each laboratory shall contain a facility for handwashing and an eye wash facility which is readily available within the work area.

(ii) An autoclave for decontamination or regulated waste shall be available.

(4) HIV and HBV production facilities shall meet the following criteria:

(i) The work areas shall be separated from areas that are open to unrestricted traffic flow within the building. Passage through two sets of doors shall be the basic requirement for entry into the work area from access corridors or other contiguous areas. Physical separation of the high-containment work area from access corridors or other areas or activities may also be provided by a double-doored clothes-change room (showers may be included), airlock, or other access facility that requires passing through two sets of doors before entering the work area.

(ii) The surfaces of doors, walls, floors, and ceilings in the work area shall be water resistant so that they can be easily cleaned. Penetrations in these surfaces shall be sealed or capable of being sealed to facilitate decontamination.

(iii) Each work area shall contain a sink for washing hands and readily available eye wash facility. The sink shall be foot, elbow, or automatically operated and shall be located near the exit door of the work area.

(iv) Access doors to the work area or containment module shall be self-closing.

(v) An autoclave for decontamination of regulated waste shall be available within or as near as possible to the work area.

(vi) A ducted exhaust-air ventilation system shall be provided. This system shall create directional airflow that draws air into the work area through the entry area. The exhaust air shall not be recirculated to any other area of the building, shall be discharged to the outside, and shall be dispersed away from occupied areas and air intakes. The proper direction of the airflow shall be verified (i.e., into the work area).

(5) *Training Requirements.*

Additional training requirements for employees in HIV and HBV research laboratories and HIV and HBV production facilities are specified in paragraph (g)(2)(ix).

(f) *Hepatitis B Vaccination and Post-Exposure Evaluation and Follow-Up.*

(1) *General.*

(i) The employer shall make available the Hepatitis B vaccine and vaccination series to all employees who have occupational exposure, and post-exposure evaluation and follow-up to all employees who have had an exposure incident.

(ii) The employer shall ensure that all medical evaluations and procedures including the Hepatitis B vaccine and vaccination series and post-exposure evaluation and follow-up, including prophylaxis, are:

(A) Made available at no cost to the employee;

(B) Made available to the employee at a reasonable time and place;

(C) Performed by or under the supervision of a licensed physician or by or under the supervision of another licensed health care professional; and

(D) Provided according to recommendations of the U.S. Public Health Service current at the time these evaluations and procedures take place, except as specified by this paragraph (f).

(iii) The employer shall ensure that all laboratory tests are conducted by an accredited laboratory at no cost to the employee.

(2) *Hepatitis B Vaccination.*

(i) Hepatitis B vaccination shall be made available after the employee has received the training required in paragraph (g)(2)(vii)(I) and within 10 working days of initial assignment to all employees who have occupational exposure unless the employee has previously received the complete Hepatitis B vaccination series, antibody testing has revealed that the employee is immune, or the vaccine is contraindicated for medical reasons.

(ii) The employer shall not make participation in a prescreening program a prerequisite for receiving Hepatitis B vaccination.

(iii) If the employee initially declines Hepatitis B vaccination but at a later date while still covered under the standard decides to accept the vaccination, the employer shall make available Hepatitis B vaccination at that time.

(iv) The employer shall assure that employees who decline to accept Hepatitis B vaccination offered by the employer sign the statement in Appendix A.

(v) If a routine booster dose(s) of Hepatitis B vaccine is recommended by the U.S. Public Health Service at a future date, such booster dose(s) shall be made available in accordance with section (f)(1)(ii).

(3) *Post-Exposure Evaluation and Follow-Up.*

Following a report of an exposure incident, the employer shall make immediately available to the exposed employee a confidential medical evaluation and follow-up, including at least the following elements:

(i) Documentation of the route(s) of exposure, and the circumstances under which the exposure incident occurred;

(ii) Identification and documentation of the source individual, unless the employer can establish that identification is infeasible or prohibited by state or local law:

(A) The source individual's blood shall be tested as soon as feasible and after consent is obtained in order to determine HBV and HIV infectivity. If consent is not obtained, the employer shall establish that legally required consent cannot be obtained. When the source individual's consent is not required by law, the source individual's blood, if available, shall be tested and the results documented.

(B) When the source individual is already known to be infected with HBV or HIV, testing for the source individual's known HBV or HIV status need not be repeated.

(C) Results of the source individual's testing shall be made available to the exposed employee, and the employee shall be informed of applicable laws and regulations concerning disclosure of the identity and infectious status of the source individual.

(iii) Collection and testing of blood for HBV and HIV serological status:

(A) The exposed employee's blood shall be collected as soon as feasible and tested after consent is obtained.

(B) If the employee consents to baseline blood collection, but does not give consent at that time for HIV serologic testing, the sample shall be preserved for at least 90 days. If, within 90 days of the exposure incident, the employee elects to have the baseline sample tested, such testing shall be done as soon as feasible.

(iv) Post-exposure prophylaxis, when medically indicated, as recommended by the U.S. Public Health Service;

(v) Counseling; and

(vi) Evaluation of reported illnesses.

(4) *Information Provided to the Health Care Professional.*

(i) The employer shall ensure that the health care professional responsible for the employee's Hepatitis B vaccination is provided a copy of this regulation.

(ii) The employer shall ensure that the health care professional evaluating an employee after an exposure incident is provided the following information:

(A) A copy of this regulation;

(B) A description of the exposed employee's duties as they relate to the exposure incident;

(C) Documentation of the route(s) of exposure and circumstances under which the exposure occurred;

(D) Results of the source individual's blood testing, if available; and

(E) All medical records relevant to the appropriate treatment of the employee including vaccination status which are the employer's responsibility to maintain.

(5) *Health Care Professional's Written Opinion.*

The employer shall obtain and provide the employee with a copy of the evaluating health care professional's written opinion within 15 days of the completion of the evaluation.

(i) The health care professional's written opinion for Hepatitis B vaccination shall be limited to whether Hepatitis B vaccination is indicated for an employee, and if the employee has received such vaccination.

(ii) The health care professional's written opinion for post-exposure evaluation and follow-up shall be limited to the following information:

(A) That the employee has been informed of the results of the evaluation; and

(B) That the employee has been told about any medical conditions resulting from exposure to blood or other potentially infectious materials which require further evaluation or treatment.

(iii) All other findings or diagnoses shall remain confidential and shall not be included in the written report.

(6) *Medical Recordkeeping.*

Medical records required by this standard shall be maintained in accordance with paragraph (h)(1) of this section.

(g) Communication of Hazards to Employees.

(1) *Labels and Signs*

    (i) Labels

        (A) Warning labels shall be affixed to containers of regulated waste, refrigerators and freezers containing blood or other potentially infectious material; and other containers used to store, transport, or ship blood or other potentially infectious materials, except as provided in paragraph (g)(1)(i)(E), (F), and (G).

        (B) Labels required by this section shall include the BIOHAZARD legend:

BIOHAZARD

        (C) These labels shall be fluorescent orange or orange-red or predominantly so, with lettering or symbols in contrasting color.

        (D) Labels required by affixed as close as feasible to the container by string, wire, adhesive, or other method that prevents their loss or unintentional removal.

        (E) Red bags or red containers may be substituted for labels.

        (F) Containers of blood, blood components, or blood products that are labeled as to their contents and have been released for transfusion or other clinical use are exempted from labeling requirements of paragraph (g).

        (G) Individual containers of blood or other potentially infectious materials that are placed in a labeled container during storage, transport, shipment, or disposal are exempted from the labeling requirement.

        (H) Labels required for contaminated equipment shall be in accordance with this paragraph and shall also state which portions of the equipment remain contaminated.

        (I) Regulated waste that has been decontaminated need not be labeled or color-coded.

    (ii) Signs.

        (A) The employer shall post signs at the entrance to work areas specified in paragraph (e), HIV and HBV Research Laboratory and Production Facilities, which shall bear the [BIOHAZARD] legend.

BIOHAZARD

(Name of the Infectious Agent)
(Special requirements for entering the area)
(Name, telephone number of the laboratory director or other responsible person)

        (B) These signs shall be fluorescent orange-red or predominantly so, with lettering or symbols in a contrasting color.

(2) *Information and Training.*

    (i) Employers shall ensure that all employees with occupational exposure participate in a training program which must be provided at no cost to the employee and during working hours.

    (ii) Training shall be provided as follows:

        (A) At the time of initial assignment to tasks where occupational exposure may take place;

        (B) Within 90 days after the effective date of the standard; and

        (C) At least annually thereafter.

    (iii) For employees who have received training on bloodborne pathogens in the year preceding the effective date of the standard, only training with respect to the provisions of the standard which were not included need be provided.

    (iv) Annual training for all employees shall be provided within one year of their previous training.

    (v) Employers shall provide additional training when changes such as modification of tasks or procedures or institution of new tasks or procedures affect the employee's occupational exposure. The additional training may be limited to addressing the new exposures created.

    (vi) Material appropriate in content and vocabulary to educational level, literacy, and language of employees shall be used.

    (vii) The training program shall contain at a minimum the following elements:

        (A) An accessible copy of the regulatory text of this standard and an explanation of its contents;

        (B) A general explanation of the epidemiology and symptoms of bloodborne diseases;

        (C) An explanation of the modes of transmission of bloodborne pathogens;

        (D) An explanation of the employer's exposure control plan and the means by which the employee can obtain a copy of the written plan;

        (E) An explanation of the appropriate methods for recognizing tasks and other activities that may involve exposure to blood and other potentially infectious materials;

        (F) An explanation of the use and limitations of methods that will prevent or reduce exposure including appropriate engineering controls, work practices, and personal protective equipment;

        (G) Information on the types, proper use, location, removal, handling, decontamination, and disposal of personal protective equipment;

        (H) An explanation of the basis for selection of personal protective equipment;

(I) Information on the Hepatitis B vaccine, including information on its efficacy, safety, method of administration, the benefits of being vaccinated, and that the vaccine and vaccination will be offered free of charge;

(J) Information on the appropriate actions to take and persons to contact in an emergency involving blood or other potentially infectious materials;

(K) An explanation of the procedure to follow if an exposure incident occurs, including the method of reporting the incident and the medical follow-up that will be made available;

(L) Information on the post-exposure evaluation and follow-up that the employer is required to provide for the employee following an exposure incident;

(M) An explanation of the signs and labels and/or color-coding required by paragraph (g)(1); and

(N) An opportunity for interactive questions and answers with the person conducting the training session.

(viii) The person conducting the training shall be knowledgeable in the subject matter covered by the elements contained in the training program as it relates to the workplace that the training will address.

(ix) Additional Initial Training for Employees in HIV and HBV Laboratories and Production Facilities. Employees in HIV or HBV research laboratories and HIV or HBV production facilities shall receive the following initial training in addition to the above training requirements:

(A) The employer shall assure that employees demonstrate proficiency in standard microbiological practices and techniques and in the practices and operations specific to the facility before being allowed to work with HIV or HBV.

(B) The employer shall assure that employees have prior experience in the handling of human pathogens or tissue cultures before working with HIV or HBV.

(C) The employer shall provide a training program to employees who have no prior experience in handling human pathogens. Initial work activities shall not include the handling of infectious agents. A progression of work activities shall be assigned as techniques are learned and proficiency is developed. The employer shall assure that employees participate in work activities involving infectious agents only after proficiency has been demonstrated.

(h) *Recordkeeping.*

(1) *Medical Records*

(i) The employer shall establish and maintain an accurate record for each employee with occupational exposure, in accordance with 29 CFR 1910.20.

(ii) This record shall include:

(A) The name and social security number of the employee;

(B) A copy of the employee's Hepatitis B vaccination status including the dates of all the Hepatitis B vaccinations and any medical records relative to the employee's ability to receive vaccination as required by paragraph (f)(2);

(C) A copy of all results of examinations, medical testing, and follow-up procedures as required by paragraph (f)(3);

(D) The employer's copy of the health care professional's written opinion as required by paragraph (f)(5); and

(E) A copy of the information provided to the health care professional as required by paragraphs (f)(4)(ii)(B), (C), and (D).

(iii) Confidentiality. The employer shall ensure that employee medical records required by paragraph (h)(1) are:

(A) Kept confidential; and

(B) Not disclosed or reported without the employee's express written consent to any person within or outside the workplace except as required by this section or as may be required by law.

(iv) The employer shall maintain the records required by paragraph (h) for at least the duration of employment plus 30 years in accordance with 29 CFR 1910.20.

(2) *Training Records*

(i) Training records shall include the following information:

(A) The dates of the training sessions;

(B) The contents or a summary of the training sessions;

(C) The names and qualifications for the persons conducting the training; and

(D) The names and job titles of all persons attending the training sessions.

(ii) Training records shall be maintained for 3 years from the date on which the training occurred.

(3) *Availability*

(i) The employer shall ensure that all records required to be maintained by this section shall be made available upon request to the Assistant Secretary and Director for examination and copying.

(ii) Employee training records required by this paragraph shall be provided upon request for examination and copying to employees, to employee representatives, to the Director, and to the Assistant Secretary in accordance with 29 CFR 1910.20.

(iii) Employee medical records required by this paragraph shall be provided upon request for examination and copying to the subject employee, to anyone having written consent of the subject employee, to the Director, and to the Assistant Secretary in accordance with 29 CFR 1910.20

(4) *Transfer of Records*

    (i) The employer shall comply with the requirements involving transfer of records set forth in 29 CFR 1910.20(h).

    (ii) If the employer ceases to do business and there is no successor employer to receive and retain the records for the prescribed period, the employer shall notify the Director, at least three months prior to their disposal and transmit them to the Director, if required by the Director to do so, within that three month period.

(i) **Dates.**

    (1) *Effective Date.* The standard shall become effective on March 6, 1992.

    (2) The Exposure Control Plan required by paragraph (c)(1) of this section shall be completed on or before May 5, 1992.

(3) Paragraph (g)(2) Information and Training and (h) Recordkeeping shall take effect on or before June 4, 1992.

(4) Paragraphs (d)(2) Engineering and Work Practice Controls, (d)(3) Personal Protective Equipment, (d)(4), Housekeeping, (e) HIV and HBV Research Laboratories and Production Facilities, (f) Hepatitis B Vaccination and Post-Exposure Evaluation and Follow-Up, and (g)(1) Labels and Signs shall take effect July 6, 1992.

Appendix A to Section 1910.1030—
Hepatitis B Vaccine Declination (Mandatory)

I understand that due to my occupational exposure to blood or other potentially infectious materials I may be at risk of acquiring Hepatitis B Virus (HBV) infection. I have been given the opportunity to be vaccinated with Hepatitis B vaccine, at no charge to myself. However, I decline Hepatitis B vaccination at this time. I understand that by declining this vaccine, I continue to be at risk of acquiring Hepatitis B, a serious disease. If in the future I continue to have occupational exposure to blood or other potentially infectious materials and I want to be vaccinated with Hepatitis B vaccine, I can receive the vaccination series at no charge to me.

Appendix C
Hepatitis B Vaccine Declination Form

Appendix A to Section 1910.1030—Hepatitis B Vaccine Declination (Mandatory)

I understand that due to my occupational exposure to blood or other potentially infectious materials I may be at risk of acquiring Hepatitis B Virus (HBV) infection. I have been given the opportunity to be vaccinated with Hepatitis B vaccine, at no charge to myself. However, I decline the Hepatitis B vaccination at this time. I understand that by declining this vaccine, I continue to be at risk of acquiring Hepatitis B, a serious disease. If in the future I continue to have occupational exposure to blood or other potentially infectious materials and I want to be vaccinated with Hepatitis B vaccine, I can receive the vaccination series at no charge to me.

Employee Signature _____

Date _____

Employer Signature _____

Date _____

Appendix D
Sample Exposure Control Plan

Note: This sample plan is provided only as a guide to assist in complying with 29 CFR 1910.1030, OSHA's Bloodborne Pathogens Standard. It is not intended to supersede the requirements detailed in the standard. Employers should review the standard for particular requirements which are applicable to their specific situation. It should be noted that this model program does not include provisions for HIV/HBV laboratories and research facilities which are addressed in section (e) of the standard. Employers operating these laboratories need to include provisions as required by the standard. Employers will need to add information relevant to their particular facility in order to develop an effective, comprehensive exposure control plan. Employers should note that the exposure control plan is expected to be reviewed at least on an annual basis and updated when necessary.

Bloodborne Pathogens Exposure Control Plan

Facility Name:_____

Date of Preparation:_____

In accordance with the OSHA Bloodborne Pathogens Standard, 29 CFR 1910.1030, the following Exposure Control Plan has been developed:

1. Exposure Determination

OSHA requires employers to perform an exposure determination concerning which employees may incur occupational exposure to blood or other potentially infectious materials. The exposure determination is made without regard to the use of personal protective equipment (i.e., employees are considered to be exposed even if they wear personal protective equipment). This exposure determination is required to list all job classifications in which all employees may be expected to incur such occupational exposure, regardless of frequency. At this facility the following job classifications are in this category:

In addition, OSHA requires a listing of job classifications in which some employees may have occupational exposure. Because not all the employees in these categories would be expected to incur exposure to blood or other potentially infectious materials, tasks or procedures that would cause these employees to have occupational exposure must also be listed in order to understand clearly which employees in these categories are considered to have occupational exposure. The job classifications and associated tasks for these categories are as follows:

Job Classification   Tasks/Procedures

2. Implementation Schedule and Methodology

OSHA also requires that this plan include a schedule and method of implementation for the various requirements of the standard. The following complies with this requirement:

Compliance Methods

Universal Precautions will be observed at this facility in order to prevent contact with blood or other potentially infectious materials. All blood or other potentially infectious material will be considered infectious regardless of the perceived status of the source individual.

Engineering and work practice controls will be used to eliminate or minimize exposure to employees at this facility. Where occupational exposure remains after institution of these controls, personal protective equipment shall also be used. At this facility the following engineering controls will be used: (list controls, such as sharps containers, etc.).

The above controls will be examined and maintained on a regular schedule. The schedule for reviewing the effectiveness of the controls is as follows: (list schedule such as daily, once/week, etc., as well as who is responsible for reviewing the effectiveness of the individual controls, such as the supervisor for each department, etc.).

Handwashing facilities are also available to the employees who incur exposure to blood or other potentially infectious materials. OSHA requires that these facilities be readily accessible after incurring exposure.

At this facility handwashing facilities are located: (list locations, such as patient rooms, procedure area, etc. If handwashing facilities are not feasible, the employer is required to provide either an antiseptic cleanser in conjunction with a clean cloth/paper towels or antiseptic towelettes. If these alternatives are used then the hands are to be washed with soap and running water as soon as feasible. Employers who must provide an alternative to readily accessible handwashing facilities should list the location, tasks, and responsibilities to ensure maintenance and accessibility or these alternatives).

After removal of personal protective gloves, employees shall wash hands and any other potentially contaminated skin area immediately or as soon as feasible with soap and water.

If employees incur exposure to their skin or mucous membranes then those areas shall be washed or flushed with water as appropriate as soon as feasible following contact.

Needles

Contaminated needles and other contaminated sharps will not be bent, recapped, removed, sheared, or purposely broken. OSHA allows an exception to this if the procedure would require that the contaminated needles be recapped or removed and no alternative is feasible and the action is required by the medical procedure. If such action is required then the recapping or removal of the needle must be done by the use of a mechanical device or a one-handed technique. At this facility recapping or removal is only permitted for the following procedures: (list the procedures and also list either the mechanical device to be used or alternatively if a one-handed technique will be used).

Containers for Reusable Sharps

Contaminated sharps that are reusable are to be place immediately, or as soon as possible, after use into appropriate sharps containers. At this facility the sharps containers are puncture resistant, labeled with a biohazard label, and are leakproof. (Employers should list here where sharps container are located as well as who has responsibility for removing sharps from containers and how often the containers will be checked to remove the sharps.)

Work Area Restrictions

In work areas where there is a reasonable likelihood of exposure to blood or other potentially infectious materials, employees are not to eat, drink, apply cosmetics or lip balm, smoke, or handle contact lenses. Food and beverages are not to be kept in refrigerators, freezers, shelves, cabinets, or on countertops or benchtops

where blood or other potentially infectious materials are present.

Mouth pipetting/suctioning of blood or other potentially infectious materials is prohibited.

All procedures will be conducted in a manner that will minimize splashing, spraying, splattering, and generation of droplets of blood or other potentially infectious materials. Methods to accomplish this goal at this facility are: (list methods, such as covers on centrifuges, usage of dental dams if appropriate, etc.).

Specimens

Specimens of blood or other potentially infectious materials will be placed in a container that prevents leakage during the collection, handling, processing, storage, and transport of the specimens.

The container used for this purpose will be labeled or color-coded in accordance with the requirements of the OSHA standard. (Employers should note that the standard provides for an exemption for specimens from the labeling/color-coding requirement of the standard provided that the facility uses Universal Precautions in the handling of all specimens and the containers are recognizable as container specimens. This exemption applies only while the specimens remain in the facility. If the employer chooses to use this exemption then it should be stated here.)

Any specimens that could puncture a primary container will be placed within a puncture-resistant secondary container. (The employer should list here how this will be carried out, e.g., which specimens, if any, could puncture a primary container, which containers can be used as secondary containers, and where the secondary containers are located at the facility.)

If outside contamination of the primary container occurs, the primary container shall be placed within a secondary container that prevents leakage during the handling, processing, storage, transport, or shipping of the specimen.

Contaminated Equipment

Equipment that has become contaminated with blood or other potentially infectious materials shall be examined before servicing or shipping and shall be decontaminated as necessary unless the decontamination of the equipment is not feasible. (Employers should list here any equipment that cannot be decontaminated before servicing or shipping.)

Personal Protective Equipment

All personal protective equipment used at this facility will be provided without cost to employees. Personal protective equipment will be chosen based on the anticipated exposure to blood or other potentially infectious materials. The protective equipment will be considered appropriate only if it does not permit blood or other potentially infectious materials to pass through or reach the employees' clothing, skin, eyes, mouth, or other mucous membranes under normal conditions of use and for the duration of time that the protective equipment will be used.

Protective clothing will be provided to employees in the following manner: (list how the clothing will be provided to employees, e.g., who has responsibility for distribution, etc., and also list which procedures would require the protective clothing and the type of protections required. This could also be listed as an appendix to this program. The employer could use a checklist as follows):

Personal Protective Equipment   Task

Gloves

Lab coat

Face shield

Clinic jacket

Protective eyewear (with solid side shield)

Surgical gown

Shoe covers

Utility gloves

Examination gloves

(list other personal protective equipment)

All personal protective equipment will be cleaned, laundered, and disposed of by the employer at no cost to employees. All repairs and replacements will be made by the employer at no cost to employees.

All garments that are penetrated by blood shall be removed immediately or as soon as feasible. All personal protective equipment will be removed before leaving the work area. The following protocol has been developed to facilitate leaving the equipment at the work area: (list where employees are expected to place the personal protective equipment on leaving the work area, and other protocols).

Gloves shall be worn where it is reasonably anticipated that employees will have hand contact with blood, other potentially infectious materials, non-intact skin, and mucous membranes. Gloves will be available from (state location and/or person who will be responsible for distributing gloves). Gloves will be used for the following procedures: (list procedures).

Disposable gloves used at the facility are not to be washed or decontaminated for re-use and are to be replaced as soon as practical when they become contaminated or as soon as feasible if they are torn, punctured, or when their ability to function as a barrier is compromised. Utility gloves may be decontaminated for re-use provided that the integrity of the glove is not compromised. Utility gloves will be discarded if they are cracked, peeling, torn, punctured, or exhibit other signs of deterioration or when their ability to function as a barrier is compromised.

Masks in combination with eye protection devices, such as goggles or glasses with solid side shield, or chin-length face shield, are required to be worn whenever splashes, spray, splatter, or droplets of blood or other potentially infectious materials may be generated and eye, nose, or mouth contamination can reasonably be anticipated. Situations at this facility that would require such protection are as follows:

The OSHA standard also requires appropriate protective clothing to be used, such as lab coats, gowns, aprons, clinic jackets, or similar outer garments. The following situations require that such protective clothing be worn:

This facility will be cleaned and decontaminated according to the following schedule: (list area and time).

Decontamination will be accomplished by using the following materials: (list the materials to be used, such as bleach solutions or EPA-registered germicides).

All contaminated work surfaces will be decontaminated after completion of procedures, immediately or as soon as feasible after any spill of blood or other potentially infectious materials, as well as at the end of the work shift if surfaces may have become contaminated since the last cleaning. (Employers should add any information concerning the use of protective coverings such as plastic wrap that keeps the surfaces free of contamination.)

All bins, pails, cans, and similar receptacles shall be inspected and decontaminated on a regularly scheduled basis (list frequency and by whom).

Any broken glassware that may be contaminated will not be picked up directly with the hands. The following procedures will be used:

Regulated Waste Disposal

All contaminated sharps shall be discarded as soon as feasible in sharps containers located in the facility. Sharps containers are located in: (specify locations of sharps containers).

Regulated waste other than sharps shall be placed in appropriate containers. Such containers are located in (specify locations of containers).

Laundry Procedures

Laundry contaminated with blood or other potentially infectious materials will be handled as little as possible. Such laundry will be placed in appropriately marked bags where it was used. Such laundry will not be sorted or rinsed in the area of use.

All employees who handle contaminated laundry will use personal protective equipment to prevent contact with blood or other potentially infectious materials.

Laundry at this facility will be cleaned at: (specify location).

(Employers should note here if the laundry is being sent off-site. If the laundry is being sent off-site, then the laundry service accepting the laundry is to be notified, in accordance with section (d) of the standard.)

Hepatitis B Vaccine

All employees who have been identified as having exposure to blood or other potentially infectious materials will be offered the Hepatitis B vaccine, at no cost to the employee. The vaccine will be offered within 10 working days of their initial assignment to work involving the potential for occupational exposure to blood or other potentially infectious materials unless the employee has previously had the vaccine or wishes to submit to antibody testing that shows the employee to have sufficient immunity.

Employees who decline the Hepatitis B vaccine will sign a waiver that uses the wording in Appendix A of the OSHA standard.

Employees who initially decline the vaccine but who later wish to have it while still covered under standard may then have the vaccine provided at no cost. (Employers should list here who has responsibility for assuring that the vaccine is offered, the waivers are signed, etc. Also the employer should list who will administer the vaccine.)

Post-Exposure Evaluation and Follow-Up

When the employee incurs an exposure incident, it should be reported to: (list who has responsibility to maintain records of exposure incident).

All employees who incur an exposure incident will be offered post-exposure evaluation and follow-up in accordance with the OSHA standard.

This follow-up will include the following:

- Documentation of the route of exposure and the circumstances related to the incident.
- If possible, the identification of the source individual and, if possible, the status of the source individual. The blood of the source individual will be tested (after consent is obtained for HIV/HBV infectivity).
- Results of testing of the source individual will be made available to the exposed employee with the exposed employee informed about the applicable laws and regulations concerning disclosure of the identity and infectivity of the source individual. (Employers may need to modify this provision in accordance with applicable local laws on this subject. Modifications should be listed here.)
- The employee will be offered the option of having their blood collected for testing of the employee's

HIV/HBV serological status. The blood sample will be preserved for up to 90 days to allow the employee to decide if the blood should be tested for HIV serological status. However, if the employee decides before that time that testing will or will not be conducted then the appropriate action can be taken and the blood sample discarded.

- The employee will be offered post-exposure prophylaxis in accordance with the current recommendations of the U.S. Public Health Service. These recommendations are currently as follows: (these recommendations may be listed as an appendix to the plan).
- The employee will be given appropriate counseling concerning precautions to take during the period after the exposure incident. The employee will also be given information on what potential illness to be alert for and to report any related experiences to appropriate personnel.
- The following person(s) has been designated to assure that the policy outlined here is effectively carried out as well as to maintain records related to this policy:

Interaction with Health Care Professionals

A written opinion shall be obtained from the health care professional who evaluates employees of this facility. Written opinions will be obtained in the following instances:

1. When the employee is sent to obtain the Hepatitis B vaccine.

2. Whenever the employee is sent to a health care professional following an exposure incident.

Health care professionals shall be instructed to limit their opinions to:

1. Whether the Hepatitis B vaccine is indicated and if the employee has received the vaccine, or for evaluation following an incident.

2. That the employee has been informed of the results of the evaluation.

3. That the employee has been told about any medical conditions resulting from exposure to blood or other potentially infectious materials. (Note that the written opinion to the employer is not to reference any personal medical information.)

Training

Training for all employees will be conducted before initial assignment to tasks where occupations exposure may occur.

Training will be conducted in the following manner:

Training for employee will include an explanation of the following:

1. the OSHA Standard for Bloodborne Pathogens

2. Epidemiology and symptomatology of bloodborne disease

3. Modes of transmission of bloodborne pathogens

4. This Exposure Control Plan, i.e., points of the plan, lines of responsibility, how the plan will be implemented, and so on

5. Procedures that might cause exposure to blood or other potentially infectious materials at this facility

6. Control methods to be used at the facility to control exposure to blood or other potentially infectious materials

7. Personal protective equipment available at this facility and who should be contacted concerning exposure to blood or other potentially infectious materials

8. Post-exposure evaluation and follow-up

9. Signs and labels used at the facility

10. Hepatitis B vaccine program at the facility

Recordkeeping

All records required by the OSHA standard will be maintained by (insert name or department responsible for maintaining records).

Dates. All provisions required by the standard will be implemented by: (insert date for implementation of the provisions of the standard).

(Employers should list here if training will be conducted using videotapes, written material, etc. Also the employer should indicate who is responsible for conducting the training.)

All employees will receive annual refresher training. (Note that this training is to be conducted within one year of the employee's previous training.)

The outline for the training material is located (list where the training materials are located.)

Appendix E
Answers to Self-Check Questions

Chapter 1

Activity 1
1. T
2. F
3. F
4. T
5. T
6. T
7. T
8. T

Chapter 2

Activity 1
1. HIV
2. HBV
3. HBV
4. HIV
5. HBV

Activity 2
Discuss with your instructor.

Chapter 3

Activity 1
1. C
2. D
3. A
4. B

Activity 2
1. C
2. C

Chapter 4

Activity 1
A. 1. T
   2. F
   3. F
   4. T
   5. T
B. 1. D
   2. C

Activity 2
Discuss with your instructor.

Chapter 5

Activity 1
1. T
2. T
3. F
4. T

Activity 2
1. C
2. B

Chapter 6

Activity 1
A. 1. F
   2. F
   3. T
   4. T
B. 1. B
   2. B
   3. C

Chapter 7

Activity 1
A. 1. F
   2. T
   3. F
   4. F
   5. T
B. 1. C
   2. A

Chapter 8

Activity 1
A. 1. B
B. 1. C
   2. A
   3. B

Chapter 9

Activity 1
1. F
2. F
3. T
4. F
5. T

Chapter 10

Activity 1
1. ✔
2.
3. ✔
4. ✔
5. ✔
6. ✔
7. ✔
8. ✔
9.

Activity 2
Discuss answers with your instructor.

Chapter 11

Activity 1
A. 1.
   2. ✔
   3. ✔
   4. ✔
   5.
   6. ✔
   7. ✔
   8. ✔
B. 1. ✔
   2. ✔
   3.
   4. ✔
   5.
   6. ✔
   7.

Chapter 12

Activity 1
1. C
2. D
3. B

Appendix F
Tuberculosis (TB)

I. Introduction

Why Is Tuberculosis Included in a Bloodborne Pathogens Manual?

This section contains information about tuberculosis (TB), an airborne disease. Since 1985, the incidence of TB in the general U.S. population has increased approximately 14 percent, reversing a 30-year downward trend. Recently, drug-resistant strains of mycobacterium tuberculosis *(M. tuberculosis)* have become a serious concern and cases of multi-drug-resistant (MDR) TB have occurred in forty states. This overview of the risks of tuberculosis exposure (although it is not a bloodborne pathogen) has been added because many employees with occupational exposure to bloodborne pathogens may potentially have occupational exposure to persons with TB disease.

Nationwide, at least several hundred health care workers (HCW) have become infected with TB and have required medical treatment after workplace exposure to TB. Twelve (12) of these HCWs have died from TB disease. In general, persons who become infected with TB have approximately a 10-percent risk for developing TB disease in their lifetimes.

What Are the 1994 CDC TB Guidelines?

The Occupational Safety and Health Administration (OSHA) has not released a standard specific to tuberculosis (as of this printing); however, the Centers for Disease Control and Prevention (CDC) has released the 1994 TB Guidelines for the protection of HCWs. OSHA believes the CDC's 1994 TB Guidelines reflect an industry recognition of the hazard as well as appropriate, widely recognized, and accepted standards of practice to be followed by employers in carrying out their responsibilities under the Act.

The CDC is not a regulatory agency. The focus of the 1994 CDC TB Guidelines is to minimize the number of HCWs exposed to *M. tuberculosis,* while maintaining optimum care of patients with active infection with *M. tuberculosis.* The guidelines can be found in the "Morbidity and Mortality Weekly Report," vol. 43, October 28, 1994. No. RR-13 Recommendations and Reports: *Guidelines for Preventing the Transmission of Mycobacterium Tuberculosis in Health-Care Facilities.*

What Is the Occupational Safety and Health Act of 1970?

OSHA is a regulatory agency. OSHA regulations are written to protect the employee from recognized hazards in the workplace. OSHA can and does enforce the worker protection by invoking the Occupational Safety and Health Act of 1970, or the General Duty Clause. The General Duty Clause (Public Law 91-596) states that "each employer shall furnish to each of his employees employment and a place of employment which are free from recognized hazards that are causing or are likely to cause death or serious physical harm to his employees: shall comply with occupational safety and health standards promulgated under this Act. Each employee shall comply with occupational safety and health standards and all rules, regulations, and orders issued pursuant to this Act which are applicable to his own actions and conduct."

Methods are available to minimize the hazards posed by employee exposure to TB. It is the employer's responsibility to see that these protections are in place and are readily available. It is your (the employee's) responsibility to utilize these protections.

Who Needs This Section?

Any employee who has potential for occupational exposure to *M. tuberculosis* needs this section. The 1994 CDC TB Guidelines specify five potentially hazardous work areas.

- Health care facilities
- Long-term care facilities for the elderly
- Homeless shelters
- Drug and treatment centers
- Correctional facilities

The following is a list of HCWs whose tasks may lead them to occupational exposure to *M. tuberculosis.*

The potential for occupational exposure is not limited to employees in these positions.

- Physicians
- Nurses
- Aides
- Home health care workers
- Dental workers
- Technicians
- Workers in laboratories and morgues
- Emergency medical service personnel
- Students
- Part-time personnel
- Temporary staff not employed by the health care facility
- Persons not directly involved with patient care, but who are potentially at risk for occupational exposure to *M. tuberculosis* (e.g., air ventilation system workers)

Meeting the General Duty Clause

The 1994 CDC TB Guidelines specify steps to be taken in order to minimize exposure to *M. tuberculosis*. In order to ensure a safe working environment and meet the OSHA General Duty Clause requirements, employers should provide the following:

1. An assessment of the risk for transmission of *M. tuberculosis* in the particular work setting

2. A protocol for the early identification of individuals with active TB

3. Training and information to ensure employee knowledge of the method of TB transmission, its signs and symptoms, medical surveillance and therapy, and site-specific protocols, including the purpose and proper use of controls (**Note:** failure to provide respirator training is citable under OSHA's general industry standard on respirators)

4. Medical screening, including pre-placement evaluation; administration and interpretation of Mantoux skin tests

5. Evaluation and management of workers with positive skin tests or a history of positive skin tests who are exhibiting symptoms of TB, including work restrictions for infectious employees

6. AFB (acid-fast bacilli) isolation rooms for suspected or confirmed infectious TB patients. These AFB isolation rooms, and areas in which high-hazard procedures are performed, should be single-patient rooms with special ventilation characteristics that are properly installed, maintained, and evaluated to reduce the potential for airborne exposure to *M. tuberculosis*.

7. Institution of Exposure Controls specific to the workplace which include the following:

- **Administrative Controls** are policies and procedures to reduce the risk of employee exposure to infectious sources of *M. tuberculosis*. An example is a protocol to ensure rapid detection of people who are likely to have an active case of TB.
- **Engineering Controls** attempt to design safety into the tools and workspace organization. An example is High Efficiency Particulate Air (HEPA) filtration systems.
- **Personal Respiratory Protective Equipment** is used by the employee to prevent exposure to potentially infectious air droplet nuclei, for example, a personal respirator.

II. Tuberculosis (TB)

What Is Tuberculosis?

- *M. tuberculosis* is the bacteria responsible for causing TB in humans.
- TB is a disease that primarily spreads from person to person through droplet nuclei suspended in the air.
- TB may cause disease in any organ of the body. The most commonly affected organ is the lung, and accounts for about 85 percent of all infection sites. Other sites may include lymph nodes, the central nervous system, kidneys, and the skeletal system.
- TB is a serious and often fatal disease if left untreated.
- Symptoms of TB include weight loss, weakness, fever, night sweats, coughing, chest pain, and coughing up blood.
- The prevalence of infection is much higher in the close contacts of TB patients than in the general population.
- There is a difference between TB infection (positive TB skin test) and TB disease.

Transmission

TB is spread from person to person in the form of droplet nuclei in the air. When a person with TB coughs, sings, or laughs, the droplet nuclei are released into the air. When another uninfected person *repeatedly* breathes in the droplet nuclei, there is a chance of their becoming infected with TB.

For an employee to develop TB infection, he or she must have close contact to a sufficient number of air droplet nuclei over a long period of time. The employee's health is also considered as contributing to the susceptibility for TB infection and the possible development of TB disease. Among the medical risk factors for developing TB are diabetes, gastrectomy (removal of the stomach), long-term corticosteroid use, immunosuppressive therapy, cancers and other malignancies, and HIV infection.

Symptoms

Symptoms of TB also occur in people with more common diseases such as a cold or flu. The difference is that the symptoms of TB disease last longer than those of a cold or flu and must be treated with prescription antibiotics. The usual symptoms of TB disease include cough, production of sputum, weight loss, loss of appetite, weakness, fever, night sweats, malaise, fatigue, and, occasionally, chest pain. Hemoptysis, the coughing up of blood, may also occur, but usually not until after a person has had TB disease for some time.

Diagnosis

TB disease is diagnosed when there is a positive AFB sputum smear, or when three successive early morning sputum specimens are cultured and there is growth of *M. tuberculosis* from at least one culture. When extrapulmonary (not in the lungs) TB is being considered, it may also be diagnosed by culture techniques. The difference is that the specimen is cultured from the site where TB is considered the cause of the infection.

III. Prevention

The 1994 CDC TB Guidelines recommend a hierarchy of controls to minimize TB transmission. These strategies are used in combination to promote workplace safety and to provide the employee with maximum protection against occupational exposure to *M. tuberculosis*. Under these guidelines, the control of TB is to be accomplished through the early identification, isolation, and treatment of persons with TB; use of engineering and administrative procedures to reduce the risk of exposure; and through the use of respiratory

Key Facts

Relationship to HIV

1. People infected with HIV and *M. tuberculosis* are at a very high risk of developing active TB. Seven to 10 percent of persons infected with both TB and HIV will develop active disease each year.
2. Extrapulmonary TB (i.e., outside the lungs) is more common in people with HIV infections.
3. Miliary TB and lymphatic TB are more common in HIV-infected people.
4. The HIV epidemic is a major contributing factor to the recent increase in cases of active TB.

protection. The CDC 1994 TB Guidelines also stress the importance of the following measures: (1) use of risk assessments for developing a written TB control plan; (2) TB screening programs for HCWs; (3) HCW training and education; and (4) evaluation of TB infection-control programs.

IV. TB Screening

Who Should Receive TB Screening?

According to the 1994 CDC TB Guidelines, HCWs are at increased risk for TB infection and should be provided with TB skin testing. This testing must be provided at no cost to employees at risk of exposure. The general population of the United States is thought to be at low risk for TB and should not be routinely tested.

Frequency of Testing

The frequency of testing is determined by the number of active cases of TB within a worksite of the facility. HCWs should receive TB skin testing prior to work in an area at increased risk for active cases of TB. A two-step TB skin testing process should be used (see What Is the Booster Effect?). Testing should be repeated each year, or more frequently for an employee assigned to a high-risk worksite or after a known exposure to a person with active TB.

What Is the TB Skin Test?

The tuberculin skin test of choice is the Mantoux test, which uses an intradermal injection of purified protein derivative (PPD). There are three strengths of PPD available; intermediate-strength (5 tuberculin units) PPD is the standard test material.

A skin test is done by injecting a very small amount of PPD just under the skin (usually the forearm is used). A small bleb (bubble) will be raised. The bleb will disappear. The injection site is then checked for reaction by your clinician about 48 to 72 hours later. If you fail to have the injection site evaluated in 72 hours, and no induration (swelling) is present, the tuberculin skin test will need to be repeated.

What Types of Reactions Occur?

Induration, the hard and bumpy swelling at the injection site, is used for determining a reaction to the PPD. Interpretation of results are best understood when the general health and risk of exposure to active TB cases are considered in the assessment. The injection site may also be red, but that does not determine a reaction to the PPD, nor indicate a positive result. We recommend that the interpretation guidelines of the

American Thoracic Society–CDC Advisory panel be used to assess the measured induration at the injection site.

What Does a Positive Result Mean?

A positive skin test means an infection with *M. tuberculosis* has occurred, but does not prove TB disease. Referral for further medical evaluation is required to determine a diagnosis of TB disease. People found to have TB disease must be provided effective treatments. These treatments would be provided to the employee by the employer if the illness was found to be work related.

Possible False Positive Results

Close contacts of a person with TB disease, who have had a negative reaction to the first skin test, should be re-tested about 10 weeks after the last exposure to the person with TB disease. The delay between tests should allow enough time for the body's immune system to respond to an infection with *M. tuberculosis*. A second test will result in a positive reaction at the injection site if an infection with *M. tuberculosis* has occurred.

Contraindications to TB Screening

If you have tested positive to the TB skin test in the past it is *not recommended* that you receive the test again. Also, pregnancy does not exclude a HCW from being tested. Many pregnant workers have been tested for TB without documented harm to the fetus. You should consult with your doctor if you are pregnant and have any questions about receiving a TB skin test.

V. Post-Exposure Reporting

What Determines an Occupational Exposure?

Occupational exposure to *M. tuberculosis* is defined as employees working in one of the five types of facilities whose workers have been identified by the CDC as having a higher incidence of TB than the general population, and whose employees have exposure defined as follows:

1. Potential exposure to the exhaled air of an individual with suspected or confirmed TB disease

2. Exposure to a high-hazard procedure performed on an individual with suspected or confirmed TB disease, which could generate potentially infectious airborne droplet nuclei

What Is the Booster Effect?

Sensitivity to the TB skin test may decrease over time, causing an initial skin test to be negative but at the same time stimulating or boosting the immune system's sensitivity to tuberculin, thereby producing a positive reaction the next time the test is given. When repeated skin testing is necessary, concern about the booster effect and the misinterpretation of skin test results can be avoided by using a two-step testing process. This is why your employer should require the two-step test as soon as you start employment. The two-step test helps to eliminate any confusion over whether an employee was infected at the worksite or was previously infected (see Recordkeeping).

Post-Exposure Evaluation and Testing

Recordkeeping
Records of employee exposure to TB, skin tests, and medical evaluations and treatment must be maintained by your employer.

Active tuberculosis disease is an illness that must be reported to public health officials. Every state has reporting requirements.

For OSHA Form 200 recordkeeping purposes, both tuberculosis infections (positive TB skin test) and tuberculosis disease are recordable. A positive skin test for tuberculosis, even on initial testing (except preassignment screening), is recordable on the OSHA 200 log because of the presumption of work-relatedness in these settings, unless there is clear documentation that an outside exposure occurred.

VI. Requirements

TB Exposure Control Plan

Employers having employees with exposure to TB shall establish a written Exposure Control Plan designed to eliminate or minimize employee exposure. This plan involves:

- Schedule and method of implementation of the control plan
- PPD testing
- Respiratory protection
- Communication of hazards to employees
- Post-exposure evaluation and follow-up
- Recordkeeping